Clean Skin
DETOX DIET

A Revolutionary Plan
to Heal Your Skin
from the Inside Out

LAUREN TALBOT, CN

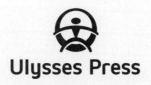

Ulysses Press

Published in the U.S. by:
Ulysses Press
P.O. Box 3440
Berkeley, CA 94703
www.ulyssespress.com

ISBN13: 978-1-61243-290-8
Library of Congress Control Number: 2013957323

Printed in Canada by Marquis Book Printing Inc.
10 9 8 7 6 5 4 3 2 1

Acquisitions Editor: Katherine Furman
Project Editor: Alice Riegert
Managing Editor: Claire Chun
Editor: Lauren Harrison
Proofreader: Elyce Berrigan-Dunlop
Index: Sayre Van Young
Cover design: what!design @ whatweb.com
Cover artwork: author shopping © Jonah Gilmore; grass background
    © varuna/shuterstock.com

Distributed by Publishers Group West

NOTE TO READERS: This book has been written and published strictly for informational and educational purposes only. It is not intended to serve as medical advice or to be any form of medical treatment. You should always consult with your physician before altering or changing any aspect of your medical treatment. Do not stop or change any prescription medications without the guidance and advice of your physician. Any use of the information in this book is made on the reader's good judgment and is the reader's sole responsibility. This book is not intended to diagnose or treat any medical condition and is not a substitute for a physician.

To Marsha, Brookie, and Kristen,
the best mother, sister, and friend a girl could ask for.
Thank you for loving me always, despite distance, diets,
and my crazy forever quest for the truth.

Contents

How to Use This Book

Hello, my beautiful readers! I could not be more excited to welcome you. These pages were created to guide you in discovering the youthful and radiant skin and complexion you desire.

In order for you to fully understand how to achieve both short-term results and long-term success, start by reading Part I carefully. It will give you valuable insight and a basic understanding of the significance of our food choices, the role of digestion, and how food and digestion play an instrumental role in our overall complexion. You will also discover everyday foods for beautiful skin and how to go about go about integrating them into your diet. Part II provides individualized guides to help start your detox program, including delicious and satiating recipes, meal plans, supplement suggestions, and skincare recommendations. If you are in a pinch for time, skip to Part II to get started, but be sure to go back to Part I for background information.

In the appendix you will find additional invaluable tools to help you grocery shop and dine out, as well as a quick reference guide for all your basic needs.

May this labor of love serve you well. You deserve to know the truth about beauty.

You were created to shine!

Introduction

With thousands of new beauty products hitting the shelves each year, it is no wonder that the beauty industry is one of the most profitable *and* crowded markets.

Products range in price as well as promise—luring us to buy into the idea of perfection in a bottle, suggesting that we can erase time and aging and cure all imperfections—under-eye circles, lines, blemishes, and various disorders of the skin—with the latest concoction or treatment. We continue our current lifestyles and cut costs on our grocery bills, opting for faster and cheaper choices, but splurge on the personal care products that carry empty promises and fake longevity.

Regardless of our expenditures in the beauty department, it is too often that we feel inadequate and unbeautiful, yet hang onto the things keeping us from achieving our goals. As you delve into these pages, the answers will unfold. May you find that what is really holding you back from being your most beautiful self is as simple as the food on your plate.

This book is designed to teach the importance of our dietary choices, how they affect our internal balance, and how we can use food to our advantage and naturally detoxify the body to deliver a beautiful and radiant complexion.

For both rapid and lasting results, I recommend reading this book from beginning to end.

Highlights

- Finally discover the beautifying secrets and solutions you have been searching for.
- Toss the expensive topical creams and prescriptions.
- Understand how your skin can be representative of what is really going on inside your body and what to do about it.
- Become empowered with the knowledge you need to get the health, body, and skin you deserve and crave.
- Watch as imperfections and signs of premature aging melt away from your skin, your mood elevates, and your body becomes effortlessly slender and tight.
- Enjoy delicious and satiating foods—old favorites and new—and never have to worry about counting calories, fat grams, or carbohydrates again.
- Acknowledge that you deserve to be and *feel* brilliant, gorgeous, talented, and fabulous. Playing small does not serve *you*, or those around you. Why suffer?
- Find that a beautiful you is much easier than you thought.

Your only regret? That you did not come across this knowledge sooner. May this book ignite your passion for natural healing and beauty, and may it make up for the years and time spent wishing you could change what you saw in the mirror.

Part I
BEFORE YOU BEGIN

CHAPTER 1

You Are What You Eat

The skin is the body's largest organ. Skin is unique in that it not only acts as a shield for our internal organs but also reflects our internal health. For instance, a zit is not merely a "clogged pore," but rather the body's way of explaining that something is not right within.

Until we find ourselves ill, it can be hard to visualize and comprehend the complexity of what is occurring on a regular basis inside the body. The skin is our looking glass. The human body is a beautifully designed powerhouse that has the ability to process the food it is given for nourishment and energy, and eliminate, to the best of its ability, the toxic waste that remains. The skin is one of the body's main channels to eliminate waste materials and toxins.

Toxic waste is removed from the body in a multitude of ways, including when we sweat, breathe, and go to the bathroom. The skin, in particular, helps us strive for internal health and balance by eliminating both natural and man-made toxins through perspiration. This is why we focus so much on our pores.

The pores, however, are not the issue. The body functions as a whole organism instead of the sum of its parts. What this means is that an imperfect complexion is not the result of poor skin, but rather a much larger issue, or internal imbalance. The outer appearance of the skin is thus brilliantly designed to help us better understand what we cannot see. Poor diet and internal and external stressors can manifest themselves as acne, dermatitis, aging, discoloration, puffiness, and lack of elasticity. Acne, or dermatitis of the skin, for instance, though emotionally debilitating, suggests a much larger problem than just a topical or bacterial issue. Disorders of the skin are the body's cry for help, and many factors can contribute to a less-than-beautiful complexion. Luckily, you have the power to alter the cards you have been dealt.

Beautiful skin starts on the inside and radiates outward. When we provide the body with more quality foods and substances than those with less nutritional value, the results are astounding. In the following chapters, you will learn how to define "quality" food.

Food Matters

A youthful, radiant, and clear complexion can only be achieved with optimal diet and digestion. The best foods for skin health, and overall health, are those that are closest to Mother Nature—foods that are whole and unprocessed. Mother Nature never intended for us to require the amount of medication that we have today. In fact, purchasing an over-the-counter pain reliever is about as easy as grabbing a soda, a bag of chips, and a candy bar. Each one of these products will be absorbed into the body and bloodstream, having some sort of effect on the body. Medications, over-the-counter remedies, antacids, prescriptions, and even vitamin supplements can create imbalances in the body by avoiding the root cause of a problem, pain, or discomfort, and masking the symptoms without treating the underlying issue. Although we like to think that we are helping our body or current predicament by swallowing a pill, we have to be aware that anything we add to the body has a reaction, good, bad, or neutral.

Like any machine, the body requires fuel to run. But unlike a car, it is a natural organism. Our food serves as our fuel, and our organs are our engine. Everything the body needs exists in nature. Man-made "nutrients" and "fortified" food groups are hardly a respectable source of nourishment. However, we are as programmed to purchase convenience in a can or box as we are to assume that beautiful skin comes in a bottle or cream.

The great news is that when we start choosing the right foods—whole, unprocessed food from nature—the human cells repair themselves, reversing disease. The end result is superior health and a beautiful, youthful, radiant, and clear complexion.

And you thought you needed that $100 face cream?

All Foods Are Not Created Equal

If you are like most of my clients, you have likely been misled to believe that you must count and measure your consumption of sugars, carbohydrates, fat, and calories. Throw these concepts out the window. Real food does not require a label. The concept of counting calories and fat grams became an important measurement only because of the processing those ingredients underwent prior to becoming packaged as new "food-like" substances. I am delighted to share with you that eating for beautiful skin will eliminate the need for you to ever count another calorie again.

What *will* matter is what type of ingredients are being used in your food. The ingredients in any packaged food are important because those ingredients, and how they are processed, will determine how well the body can utilize the food for energy and beauty, and also how easily it will be able to eliminate the remaining waste.

If food is properly and completely digested, assimilated, broken down, and then eliminated, we need not worry about the calories, or lack thereof. Real, plant-based foods that are closest to their origin in nature are the most nutrient-dense, hydrating, and nourishing foods that we can consume. In addition to their attractive nutrient profile, they are also quick to nourish and quick to be eliminated. If a nutrition label is lengthy and contains ingredients that you cannot quickly decipher (let alone pronounce), drop it. Both your waistline and your skin do not care if a manufactured food source has zero calories and sugar if it cannot be utilized for beauty and health.

The body is an incredible mechanism. It finds energy in unfit and processed foods. However, it does not do so without consequence. The body only finds *sustainable*, life-force building, and beautifying energy in foods that are unprocessed and living. Fruits, vegetables, greens, and unprocessed grains are nutrient-dense and more easily digested, providing vitamins, minerals, and antioxidants essential to healthy skin.

The body also happens to be quite clever. The skin is a back-up organ for toxic waste removal. Unwanted byproducts that the liver and kidneys could not efficiently neutralize can be redirected for removal via the pores. This process is an effective protective mechanism. For instance, it recognizes that acne, though socially debilitating and aesthetically unappealing, is much less deadly than liver disease. The body will attempt to protect the most vital of organs first, which is why skin disorders are among the first visible signs of an imbalanced diet.

Digestion and Elimination

Digestion begins in the stomach and upper part of the small intestine. After food leaves the stomach, it is passed on to the small intestine, where the body extracts nutrients and passes the remaining waste to eventually be eliminated. Nutrient absorption does not occur in the stomach, but in the small intestine. This is important because the length of time a meal requires for digestion in the stomach determines how long our body must wait before it can begin to utilize the vitamins, minerals, and nutrients it requires and values. It also determines the rate at which we accumulate excess wastes. Waste increases the rate at which we age, causing deterioration of the skin: uneven tone, loss of elasticity, puffiness, and dull, lifeless color.

A meal with a lengthy transit time, from stomach to small intestine, will remain in the body far longer than intended. The aftermath of a slow-digesting meal is similar to leaving the kitchen trash out for too long. It will smell of rot and decay. The longer food sits, the more time it has to ferment, decay, and create toxic waste for the blood to absorb. These toxins will then be eliminated through various organs, including the skin. Meals with quick transit times will promote good digestion, cleanse the cells and blood, and leave the body with little waste residue.

The digestive tract is a whopping 25 feet long, with the small intestine representing 20 feet, and the larger, wider intestine (the colon), representing 5. Why is this relevant? The food we ingest has to make it through 25 feet of intestine before it can be efficiently eliminated through feces.

Depending on your daily routine and diet, this means you should be visiting the restroom approximately two or three times a day (not two or three times a week!). It's an unladylike topic, but your bowels and bathroom habits are a telltale sign of how your body is responding to the foods and beverages you nourish it with. A common thread in my practice when evaluating a client with a skin disorder is insufficient digestion. This is generally matched with issues like irregularity, constipation, and a mild case of some type of inflammatory bowel syndrome.

Unfortunately, because discussing bathroom habits can be rather uncomfortable for everyone, bowel movements and digestion are often overlooked or just "solved" with medication or laxatives. With a proper diet, you don't require medication to have a healthy, working digestive and eliminatory system.

Enzymes and Digestion

Enzymes are biologically active substances, produced by a living organism. An enzyme acts as a catalyst for change, or specific reaction in the body. Enzymes are required for cellular activity and metabolism. In other words, we need these substances—without them, there would be no life. There are three types of enzymes:

- **Metabolic Enzymes**—these enable us to see, hear, breathe, move, think, and feel.
- **Digestive Enzymes**—these enzymes are created by the body, primarily the small intestine and pancreas, but also the stomach and saliva glands, in order to break down the food we eat and turn it into usable nutrients and waste. Many people take digestive enzyme supplements to enhance sluggish digestion, which especially increases with "premature aging."
- **Food Enzymes**—these are the active enzymes that are found in fresh, uncooked foods. Ideally these "raw" foods have enough enzymes to be able to digest the food itself without having to utilize the body's reserve of digestive enzymes, thus avoiding excess stress on the body.

Digestive enzymes and the food enzymes found in raw foods enable us to digest and assimilate the foods that we eat, readily absorb the nutrients, and get rid of the waste efficiently. Foods that contain these life-building enzymes are whole plant foods. When we enjoy diets that are void of food enzymes (meaning most cooked foods, excluding lightly steamed vegetables), the digestive system has to work harder to break down the food, absorb the nutrients, and excrete the waste. In our culture where meat is a staple product and there is a fast food joint and a vending machine at every corner, we are eating foods that are not only void of enzymes, but also void of nutrients altogether.

In other words, the Standard American Diet places extra stress on an otherwise beautiful system while living plant foods can facilitate the digestive process, ideally allowing the body to absorb more nutrients, with reduced accumulation.

If we nourish the body with life-generating greens, fruits, and vegetables and limit (and ultimately eliminate) the amount of life-deteriorating foods we ingest, the body can focus on beauty. If our diet is the opposite of beautiful, we force the body to devote excess energy to digestion and the elimination of toxic waste. This diversion steals our enzymes, radiance, youth, and health.

pH and Beautiful Skin

Beautiful skin starts from within and radiates outward. Just as the ideal complexion is balanced—not too oily or too dry—the ideal internal state of our health relies on balance too.

This balance is referred to as our body's "potential of hydrogen," more commonly known as pH. pH is a measure of the acidity or alkalinity of a solution on a scale of 0–14, where 0 represents the most acidic and 14 the most alkaline. If a solution is said to have a pH of 7, it is neutral. Battery acid has a pH of about 1, whereas drain cleaner has a pH of around 14.

Bodily fluids, including blood, saliva, and urine, strive to maintain a relatively neutral and slightly alkaline pH (about 7.3–7.5). Every metabolic process relies on the alkalinity of these bodily fluids to function optimally. At this level, cells are capable of regenerating and healing far beyond the power of what any fancy skin care regimen or ointment can do for them. Acidity in the body pulls the body's focus from regeneration to "waste removal." This demands more of the organs and creates unwanted stress, meaning that when the body is in an acid state, the result is stress and toxicity. Toxins are eliminated through the skin and cause acne.

Many factors, like everyday stressors and the Standard American Diet, are highly acid-forming and offset our pH. Acidity is a breeding ground for disease and bacteria, while in a neutral or slightly alkaline environment, bacteria will not flourish. When the body is alkaline, for instance, it is not capable of catching a cold from the person who sneezes nearby, as the bacteria have nothing to fuel their reproductive success. In other words, if no one is home, if there is nothing to eat, bacteria are forced to move on or die out.

Because we cannot control every aspect of our life, our dietary choices are one of the easiest opportunities for us to balance the body's pH. Eating an alkaline diet does not need to be complicated. Processed and refined carbohydrates (white flour and wheat flour), alcohol, processed sugars and most sugar substitutes, animal products, dairy, and gluten are acid-forming foods. Whole, plant-based foods that are closest to their origin in nature, are more alkaline. The deeper the green and the closer to nature, the more alkaline a food is. A diet low in acid-forming foods and rich in fruits and especially dark leafy greens and vegetables creates the ideal environment for radiant skin. For a more thorough list of alkaline and acidic foods see "The pH of Common Foods" on page 196.

Over time, an acidic diet will corrode the intestinal piping system and tissues and impair the body's ability to absorb nutrients and function optimally. Not only do acid-forming foods create a pH imbalance, but they also slow metabolism and create the perfect environment for bacteria and disease to thrive. Acidity in the body thus becomes highly damaging to the vital organs and skin.

Tests exist to check your body's pH. These, however, are quite unnecessary. The body functions as a whole organism and not the sum of its parts. In other words, if the skin is suffering, we already know that the body is not in balance.

OTHER FACTORS THAT CAN AFFECT pH

A few common examples of external factors that lower our pH are prescription medications, recreational drugs, alcohol, stress, pollution, negative relationships, insufficient sleep, and overexercise.

Prescription medications and recreational drugs offset our pH by chemically altering our internal environment to mask, or "treat," specific issues. They can also affect the way our body digests and assimilates nutrients from our food, causing issues such as constipation, diarrhea, nutritional imbalances, and malnutrition. Depending on the type of medication, prescription medications can be damaging to the good bacteria in the body. These good bacteria, commonly referred to as probiotics, help in the digestive process and the elimination of waste. Without them, the body cannot defend itself from intrusive viruses, parasites, and bacteria, which directly and indirectly degrade the skin and weaken the immunity. Other medications such as oral contraceptives or corticosteroids, used to treat asthma, can create the perfect environment for toxic yeasts and fungi like candida (also referred to as "thrush" when located orally) to colonize and reproduce. I often see candida-related issues in my practice, especially when a client is dealing with acne or itchy rashes. Candida is so relevant to the skin it will be discussed in greater length in "pH, Antibiotics, Yeast Imbalances, and the Immune System" on page 21.

Stressors from work, relationships, and daily life can also be damaging, as can overexercise, overexertion of energy, and insufficient sleep. We all feel the effects of these stressors at different points in our lives and sometimes daily. These external factors affect the way our body releases hormones into the blood, as well as how vital organs function, for example causing increased heart rate, restricted breathing and decreased flow of oxygen, constipation, and indigestion.

Often underestimated, sleep is extraordinarily healing. It is one of the only opportunities for the body to focus on rest and cell regeneration instead of external stressors and food consumption. Strive to give yourself eight hours of rest each night. If you have trouble sleeping, a plant-based magnesium supplement can be relaxing, restful, and cleansing. Magnesium also happens to be one of the most alkaline minerals in the body. Although commonly thought to help one fall asleep, alcohol can hinder deep, restful sleep. Other common habits that affect and disrupt our sleep are television and computer use before bed, caffeine, sugar, heavy and miscombined meals, and other processed and difficult-to-digest foods. An acceptable dessert in this lifestyle is dark chocolate. That being said, chocolate contains theobromine, a stimulating substance similar to caffeine. This can also affect one's ability to fall asleep. If you are sensitive to caffeine or prone to anxiety, avoid eating chocolate at least three hours before bed or opt out altogether.

Common Skin Disorders

Some of the most common skin ailments discussed in the beauty departments of many stores are premature aging, inflammation, and acne. Though distinctly different, they are in fact largely associated and a product of internal imbalance. Let's take a deeper look at the most common threats our skin sees.

PREMATURE AGING

In our Western society of low-grade nutrition, we have come to expect our bodies to wrinkle and sag at any time during our maturity. We are learning to expect these signs of aging way before our prime. Premature aging is described as a loss of elasticity, or resistance, in our skin; this includes wrinkles, deep laugh lines, darkness around the eyes, looking tired, and a lack of color in the skin or discoloration. It also means we trade our baby soft, supple, and dewy skin for a leathery, rough, and "dried-out" exterior. Regardless, as a result of our lifestyle and diet, we look older than we should.

INFLAMMATION

This broad term is used to describe many common disorders of the skin. Often described as reddened, swollen, hot, and painful, inflammation is what occurs when the skin produces a variety of inflammatory hormones in response to a triggered stimulus—something the body has learned it does not like. These hormones hook up with other inflammatory hormones and can activate nerve cells, dilate blood vessels, and send immune cells to the skin, producing inflammation.

Inflammation can be separated into two categories: acute and chronic. Acute inflammation is when the skin reacts adversely to an allergen, radiation, or a chemical irritant. The immediate removal of this irritant usually results in the elimination of the adverse reaction. Acute inflammation can generally last between seven and fourteen days, and without repeated exposure causes little to no permanent damage to skin tissues.

Chronic inflammation of the skin is the damage caused by sustained reactions from within the skin itself. Although inflammation is an immune response designed to keep foreign invaders and bacteria out of the body, when the body is in a state of chronic inflammation caused by continuous exposure to unwanted stimuli (like poor diet, overexercise, stress, chemicals, drugs and alcohol, synthetics, and pharmaceuticals), the result is serious tissue damage to the skin. Inflammation comes in all shapes and sizes. Inflammatory disorders of the skin include rashes, rosacea, eczema, and psoriasis, but also aging and acne.

Rashes

Rashes are generally itchy and pinkish-red, and can be caused by coming into contact with environmental factors such as cosmetics, perfume, and fragrances. It can be common to develop a rash from particular metals in jewelry. Rashes can also become present after the consumption of a particular food. If one has candida, for instance, they might become itchy and develop a rash after the consumption of too much fruit.

Eczema

Considered a genetic disorder, eczema causes the skin around the elbows and behind the knees to become various degrees of itchy, red, and flaky.

Psoriasis

Also considered a genetic disorder, psoriasis is the buildup of excess skin tissue that becomes inflamed, scaly, swollen, and itchy. It can spread from the hands to the joints, limbs, and to the trunk of the body.

Rosacea

Rosacea is characterized as consistent flushing of the cheeks, eyelids, and nose.

Acne

Considered a result of clogged pores, acne is commonly associated with uncleanliness. Acne is typically located on the face, shoulders, back, and chest. There are several common terms associated with acne:

Pimple: Characterized as a pink or red bump that can appear alone or in a cluster. Pimples of this nature are generally surrounded by inflammation, or redness of the skin, making them look all the more unpleasant.

Blackhead: A plugged-up and widened hair follicle or pore that is darkened by oxidation.

Whitehead: The same as a blackhead, only the bacteria is trapped inside what appears to be a white bubble.

Cystic and Nodulocystic Acne: These most severe forms of acne result in large and severely inflamed lumps that either harden or can appear to contain fluid. Severe acne can be extremely uncomfortable, painful, and form deep within the skin. Lumps of this nature can take a long time to vanish.

Skin Conditions and Food Sensitivities

Most of us have trouble connecting the dots between what we eat and how we look because the appearance of our skin is not generally immediately affected by our choices. It could take years of unfit food consumption before our internal inflammation and imbalance "catches up to us" and we start to notice more severe discomforts and intolerances to something we "used to eat all the time."

When the intestines are inflamed, the body becomes more sensitized to food and will react in a number of ways. Although rarely taken into account, food sensitivities can result in or contribute to acne and create or worsen various topical skin disorders. It can be beneficial to keep a record of what is being consumed to help pinpoint trigger foods. Depending on the food, "allergies" of this sort are generally only temporary until the inflammation is reduced and eliminated.

Certain plant foods that may trigger allergic-like reactions over a period of time are generally those higher in protein, like avocados, nuts, coconuts, and grains, especially foods with gluten, to name just a few. There are also foods that may innocently cause irritation, like eggplant and mango. Be on guard if you notice any irritation one to seven days after consuming a food, especially when the eruption takes place around the mouth.

You may not notice that animal proteins cause reactions because not all food sensitivities trigger noticeable or immediate responses when consumed. Although I have had several clients observe a direct correlation to a skin issue and chicken consumption, the majority of my clients will only notice a significant difference in their skin after minimizing or eliminating animal products. This is simply because animal products are acid-forming, and help to create the inflammation triggering a "leaky gut." It is this leaking gut, caused by unfit foods, and/or an imbalance of acidity in the body, that causes us to develop "allergies" or "sensitivities" to certain otherwise harmless foods. I have had several clients come to me after testing positive for beneficial foods like garlic or onions, but the rest of their diet is not in balance. In other words, it is not the garlic or onion that are to blame, but rather the other unfit substances causing us to become irritated by normally beneficial foods.

Unfit foods consistently cause adverse effects on the body and can lead to specific skin disorders.

REFINED SUGARS

Refined ingredients like those found in packaged and shelf-stable foods are broken down into quickly metabolized simple sugars. This sugar leaves an acid residue in the body. That acidic state can create and worsen inflammation and feed the bacteria and yeasts like candida. This inflammation can become a catalyst for rapid aging.

ALCOHOL

Alcohol is high in sugar and very yeast-forming, which contributes to a yeast imbalance in the body and triggers acne. It's also highly acid-forming and lowers the body's pH. This accelerates the aging process by dehydrating and thinning the skin. Healthy skin is noticeably more supple and "dewy."

Alcohol consumption also contributes to inflamed, acne-prone skin because it stresses the liver (and kidneys), which has to process the alcohol. The liver uses the skin as its backup organ for the removal of toxins. When the internal organs are overloaded with toxins, the result is bloat and puffiness around the eyes and face.

STIMULANTS

Stimulants are a class of drugs that stimulate brain activity. They range from the commonly accepted and widely used stimulants like caffeine (found in coffee, tea, soda, and energy drinks), theobromine (chocolate), and nicotine (cigarettes), but also include amphetamines, cocaine, and prescription drugs.

Like alcohol, stimulants like cocoa and coffee can have a diuretic effect on the body and cause dehydration. And even these lesser of evils are acid-forming and can stress the liver as well as the adrenal glands. The regular consumption of stimulants can skew the body's pH balance, weaning the immune system and creating a place for acne-causing bacteria to thrive. Additionally, overworked and stressed adrenal glands will create hormonal imbalances that accelerate aging.

ANIMAL PRODUCTS

Found in abundance in products such as milk, cheese, and meat, hormones affect our emotions, moods, stress levels, and menstrual cycles. All of these contribute to inflammation, toxicity, and internal imbalance. Hormone-triggered imbalances are catalysts for acne-causing bacteria to flourish, as well as for rapid aging and degeneration. Hormones are given to animals in order to enable them to unnaturally produce more milk or speed the rate of their growth and development. This decreases the length of time an animal needs to be raised and enhances its worth, while becoming an indirect detriment to our own hormonal system.

Other Factors That Can Cause Skin Disorders

It is commonplace to blame hormonal imbalances as reasons for our skin issues. This internal balance is of paramount importance for a youthful complexion and clear skin. Additionally, exercise, often considered a solution for weight loss, can also play a considerable role in our overall complexion.

HORMONES AND INTERNAL IMBALANCE

The endocrine system influences almost every cell, organ, and function in our bodies. It is largely responsible for our mood, growth and development, reproductive organs, and sexual function, as well as the break down and assimilation of nutrients in the body. The goal of the endocrine system is to maintain a balance that promotes our well-being. It reacts to hormonal changes in the blood by secreting hormones when levels are low and halting production when levels are high. The endocrine glands work to maintain this balance.

However, because our diets are so out of tune with our bodies' needs and the demands of our organs, especially as we age, our endocrine systems struggle to maintain that balance. Thus we suffer from issues commonly attributed to a decrease in hormone levels like low sex drive, trouble regulating the body's temperature, anxiety, joint pain, sleeplessness, vaginal dryness, constipation, hair loss, and drastic changes in the skin. As a prescription to treat hormonal imbalances, estrogen and synthetic estrogens are commonly supplemented to replace the natural decrease women experience with age. Conversely, lower levels of estrogen do not always indicate a disorder, but are a natural life progression.

Similarly, the birth control pill is a common prescription for acne. The pill works by supplying synthetic forms of progesterone and estrogen to prevent the natural processes of ovulation and menstruation. Its intended use for treating acne is to alter hormonal shifts in the body that can be linked to breakouts. Although acne can be caused by hormonal imbalances, the hormonal imbalance is only a symptom of a much larger issue: nutritional imbalance. Because the birth control pill does not address those nutritional deficiencies, the introduction of synthetic hormones to the body can create other medical issues, including anxiety and depression—two disorders that can contribute to and worsen stress levels, inflammation, and acne.

Additionally, estrogen stimulates the production of glycogen, which feeds the vaginal pathogens that weaken immunity and contribute to breakouts. Shifts in estrogen are also largely responsible for cravings that feed these undesirable bacteria and yeast. For more information on contraceptives and skin, see "Women, Candida, and Contraceptives" on page 23.

WEIGHT AND EXERCISE

Stored toxins reside in the fatty tissue of the human body. Toxins will either be stored internally or eliminated. If eliminated, the result may be acne. Hence, someone with a slim physique can have a blemished complexion. When one has a lower BMI (Body Mass Index), *and* an imbalanced diet (or pH), there are fewer places for these toxins to be kept. A rigorous exercise program that is not backed up with a sufficiently alkaline diet will result in premature aging and wrinkles.

In fact, a good workout regimen, although beneficial in many respects, does not replace a poor diet. Many of us do not realize the short- and long-term impact our food and "energy sources" have on our body, beyond our taste buds, stomach, and a summation of expended calories and fat grams. The hard truth is: "calories in" does not equal "calories out." We cannot expect to "burn off" a latte and a muffin at the gym and not suffer consequences elsewhere down the line. Exercise and diet are not interchangeable when it comes to our health and beauty. There is no "out of sight, out of mind."

Not all toxins from waste accumulation will immediately result in poor skin because toxins can be stored in the fatty tissue of the body to *prevent* them from being in continuous circulation or damaging vital organs. Weight is not an ultimate indicator of our internal health. The body has different ways of manifesting an internal imbalance. It is for this reason that a trim person with low body fat may sometimes suffer from premature aging, wrinkles, and acne. In fact, a very fit person with an insufficient diet or too much stress on the liver and kidneys may appear to age more quickly than a heavier, less fit person. With fewer fat cells, slender people have less room to store toxins. Do not be quick to assume that you merely need a topical skin treatment or hormonal pill just because you are thin, active, and burning calories. On the flip side, being overweight is not desirable either because, good skin or not, it means the body is carrying around more stored waste and toxins.

pH, Antibiotics, Yeast Imbalances, and the Immune System

Within the body there exist little armies of antibodies and white blood cells. These microscopic armies defend the body from enemy substances that are looking to harm or weaken it. When the immune system is strong, these armies are able to recognize and then deactivate, kill, or eliminate the enemies before they are capable of causing the body damage. The antibody armies create a protective barrier, lining the delicate mucous membranes that line the interior cavities and passageways of the body. Directly below the mucous membrane exist mucus-secreting glands. In order to protect the membranes, these glands secrete a coating of sticky mucus that traps toxins and prevents them from penetrating farther into the body and contaminating the blood.

When toxins, yeasts, and other such enemies—known as antigens—attempt to invade the mucous membrane, the antibodies come to the body's defense, forbidding the antigens to cause destruction. When diet and lifestyle are compromised, the antibodies are weakened and antigens make their way into the bloodstream. When the body is undernourished and in an acidic state, detrimental incidences occur: bacteria and pathogens are allowed to multiply at an exponential rate, and the organs are forced to work overtime to rid the body of unwanted substances. In this compromised state, the body ages more quickly, is more susceptible to disease, and the skin becomes dull, congested, and blemished.

Many antibiotics are considered effective in treating bacterial and common infections because they eliminate symptoms caused by an overgrowth of bad bacteria. They do so by destroying bad organisms or preventing them from reproducing. But because antibiotics are considered unnatural and acid-forming, they lower our body's pH. This acidic state helps to create an ideal environment for toxic yeasts like candida and other bad bacteria to flourish as they also destroy the internal flora, or healthy probiotics, in the body. I often refer to probiotics as our body's little army of "gardeners." Every garden has some weeds, as every body harbors some bad bacteria and yeasts. A good gardener manages the weeds to prevent them from taking over the garden. Our healthy flora—probiotics—prevent bad bacteria and toxic yeasts from multiplying like a gardener tending to their flower beds. When yeasts such as candida are allowed to multiply, they release toxins. These toxins circulate throughout the body and further depress the immune system. This issue becomes recurring in individuals that continuously find themselves on a round of antibiotics.

In addition to antibiotics, birth control pills, cortisone, and other drugs like prednisone, corticosteroids, and acne medication stimulate yeast growth. The unfortunate irony is, dermatological medications and birth control pills are commonly prescribed to heal skin issues, especially acne. Though these medications fight to kill off the toxins that weaken the immune system and generate skin issues and allergies, they also deplete the body's reservoir of friendly bacteria and can create an acidic environment for those same bad bacteria to return. Without the help of friendly bacteria, the body does not have the ability to resist the colonization of harmful yeasts, and thus it becomes an endless battle as the body attempts to rid itself of unwanted toxins.

Candida, or candidiasis, is used to describe a number of syndromes associated with toxic yeast colonization. Superficial infections associated with candida presence include oral thrush, common in infants and individuals on prescriptive asthma medication, vaginitis, jock-itch, and skin disorders, including rashes and acne. Although toxic to the human body, candida is likely present, to some extent, in almost every human body, but limited in growth by a strong immune system, healthy bacteria, and an alkaline diet. However, our Western lifestyle has allowed it to become a root cause for disease and, more specifically, a major factor in the appearance of our skin.

If you are on antibiotics, and other hormonal, or prescription medications, consult with your doctor, and/or holistic practitioner about more natural solutions to return the body to its naturally alkaline state of harmony and balance. The Clear Skin Detox plan suggested in this book is a naturally detoxifying diet of whole plant-based, alkaline foods, designed to reduce and eliminate inflammation and rebalance the normal functioning of the body, reducing and even eliminating the need for pharmaceuticals and over-the-counter remedies. When I work with a client, the end goal is to transform their skin and health with their lifestyle and dietary choices, internal cleansing (which will be visited in a separate chapter), and plant-based supplementation.

• • • •

WOMEN, CANDIDA, AND CONTRACEPTIVES

Women in particular seem more susceptible to a common cause of skin problems associated with candida. Why women? In general, yeasts thrive in warm, damp, dark places and, therefore, are commonly abundant in the digestive tract and vaginal area.

Other factors (exclusive to women) such as hormonal changes during adolescent years, pregnancy, menopause, and birth control pills also contribute to candida's growth.

Medications that affect our hormones, like the birth control pill, patch, or ring, are often prescribed to help treat skin disorders. However, these medications use synthetically designed (i.e., man-made) hormones, estrogen and progesterone, to inhibit what the body was *naturally* built to do—ovulate and cleanse through menstruation (shedding of the uterine lining). Birth control pills also change the lining of the female reproductive organs, making it inhospitable for new life. Granted, bringing new life into the world is not on every woman's agenda, but a healthy and balanced body should be otherwise prime for generating new life regardless. For this reason, I only suggest nonhormonal forms of contraceptives, such as condoms.

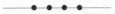

CRAVINGS AND YEAST IMBALANCES

Aside from stressors, medication, hormonal imbalances, and poor nutrition habits, candida (a living yeast, or fungi, itself) feeds off of a particular diet very common in women, who are more susceptible to candida than men: one that is in high in sugar, vinegar, refined carbohydrates (aka carbs), foods containing yeast, pickled foods, and molds and fungi. The most common foods in our diet that are highly susceptible to mold are cheeses, mushrooms, melons, tomatoes, malt, dried fruit, peanuts, and nuts. In this dietary "environment," healthy bacteria are unable to protect against the reproduction and colonization of the "bad bacteria," and the body suffers.

COMMON SYMPTOMS OF CANDIDA

- Gas or bloat after eating fruit
- Frequent indigestion, constipation, diarrhea, etc., after meals
- Acne (mild to severe), or frequent breakouts
- Rashes, or dermatitis of the skin
- Cravings for sugar, "carbs," and breads
- Low energy
- Irritability, depression, or anxiety
- Foggy or clouded thinking
- Recurring yeast or vaginal infections

Luckily, candida is something that can be treated and managed with diet. Though every individual may have candida in varying degrees, a "candida-free" diet is something that any and every individual can benefit from.

With the reduction (and sometimes absolute elimination) of foods that candida is attracted to, especially refined grains, processed sugars, fruit sugars, alcohol, oils, and heated fats and animal proteins, you will discover increased energy, optimum digestion, and a youthful, radiant, and *clear* complexion all without the assistance of (oral or topical) medication. Read on for more specific dietary recommendations.

CHAPTER 2

Foods to Avoid and Their Alternatives

It bears repeating here that the digestive tract, or specifically the small and large intestines, are approximately 25 feet of spongy tissue. Nutrients are absorbed through this tissue and into the bloodstream, which transfers them to the essential organs so they can be used for energy and nourishment. Without proper nutrition, the organs do not receive the raw vitamins and minerals they require to live a long and healthy life, and slowly the body begins to deteriorate. If one organ begins to suffer, the other organs are compromised as well, including the largest and most visible one—the skin.

Remember, foods are not created equally. As far as the body is concerned, there is a definite hierarchy. The ingredients in the vast majority of packaged foods are generally processed beyond recognition and then "fortified" and "enriched" with nutrients that have been removed during the production process. These foods are then pumped with artificial ingredients that add cheap flavor and generally contribute to the product's unnaturally long shelf life. While these factors may seem practical, and even beneficial, artificial ingredients and added preservatives help no one but those in the Big Food industry.

When production is cheap and shelf life is long, Big Food rakes in the big bucks by creating popularly addicting foods that they can inexpensively sell by the dozen. This type of "profit" would be fine if it did not come at a high cost to those consuming it. While this fast food and snack food may seem cheaper, the savings are only up front.

Each year as the medical bills increase exponentially, so do the rates for obesity, high cholesterol, and diabetes, to name just a few. In addition to this massive health crisis, the exponential and potential growth of mass-marketed weight-loss, detox, and beauty products is increasing just as fast. When you invest money in the food you fuel your body with, you save money at the pharmacy, beauty counter, and healthcare provider's office. You also save time that would be spent singing the blues and avoiding the mirror.

If we are to improve the skin, we must start by eliminating foods that slow digestion and/or leave behind unwanted residue after they are used as "fuel" for the body.

The standard Western diet and lifestyle is high in cheaply processed, artificial, and chemically treated ingredients, as well as dairy and meats. These foods are not easy for the body to digest, process, and eliminate. The result is that food sits in the intestines longer than it was intended. As food (waste, at this point) sits, it putrefies, ferments, decays, and can cause inflammation of the intestines and the rest of the body.

If we reduce and eliminate the following, the result is clearer skin in as little as a few days.

Foods to Avoid for Radiant Skin

MILK

Every year, the average American consumes about 600 pounds of dairy. Despite this alarming number, dairy is a leading cause of digestive issues and skin disorders. Aside from processed and refined products, milk and dairy products are one of the first "foods" to eliminate from your diet. Reasons to avoid milk:

Milk is high in sugar. This simple sugar is known as *lactose*. In order to digest lactose, we must have the enzyme *lactase*. People who are lactose-intolerant are lacking this enzyme. What is fascinating about a mother's milk is that it contains *both* lactose and lactase. For this reason, most babies are able to comfortably enjoy their mother's milk. In other words, a mother's milk (cow, human, cat, dog, etc.) is a package deal and designed for its own offspring. A cow's milk was designed for a baby cow, not a human infant— or a grown adult, for that matter. We are the only living beings in the animal kingdom that not only drink milk after infancy, but also drink another living creature's milk.

Milk is intended to build the skeletal structure during development. The offspring no longer needs its mother's milk when its body is developed enough to absorb and assimilate the whole foods that nature intended.

Cow's milk is intended to nourish a baby cow. Cow's milk nourishes and supports the growth from an 85-pound calf to a 1,500-pound cow. As Dr. Norman W. Walker, one of the pioneers for understanding digestive health, wrote in 1995, "Cow's milk is intended to double the weight of the calf in 6 to 8 weeks, whereas a child requires 6 to 7 months to double its weight."

Milk contains casein. Casein is among the slowest-to-digest proteins. All animal milks contain casein, but a cow's milk contains 300 percent more casein than a human mother's milk, making it unfit for human consumption.

Milk is pasteurized. When milk is pasteurized, it is heated to a temperature that destroys the majority of bacteria that could exist in unpasteurized milk. Cows that are raised in inorganic settings are generally a breeding ground for bacteria and all sorts of pathogens. However, pasteurization also destroys good bacteria (probiotics), vitamins, and minerals. For this reason, we usually see milk on our grocers' shelves exclaiming, "fortified with (<u>fill in the blank</u>)." Milk products are fortified because the majority of vitamins and minerals were destroyed during the heating process, and the milk industry needs to add something back to the milk in order to make it "nutritious."

Milk is fortified with an *animal* source of vitamin A. Vitamin A from a plant source, such as a carrot, is very beneficial to the skin. Animal sources of vitamin A are unbeneficial, acidic, and linked to deterioration of the skeletal structure

Milk has harmful additives. There are also other additives hidden in inorganic milk products, including but not limited to hormones and antibiotics. These additives are extremely detrimental to the skin, digestion, and health. This can also overstimulate mucus production, making milk very congesting.

Removing cow dairy from your diet, particularly as a beverage, will produce both immediate and long-lasting improvements in the skin. If using milk in your tea, coffee, or cereal is an integral part of your diet, it may be challenging to cut it out immediately without replacement. It is important to not feel overly restricted, which can make any new regimen more difficult to follow and stick with. Try these alternatives instead:

Milk Alternatives

Almond, hazelnut, sunflower, and coconut milk (preferably unsweetened, not just "sugar-free"). You can also easily make your own nut and seed milks with a nut milk bag, purchased online. We will not cover this topic in this book. Do not use rice or soy as a milk alternative.

CHEESE

Cheese is another commonly consumed dairy product that creates digestive discomfort and skin disorders. Many of its negative aspects are the same as those of cow's milk, but it also comes with its own health drawbacks.

Simply put, "cheese" is the broad term given to a diverse group of milk products that have been created by curdling the casein protein in milk. Cheese is most frequently made from cow's milk, but is also often made from the milk of buffalo, sheep, and goats as well. Some of these options make better choices than cow's milk cheese. In a nutshell, all cheeses are composed of milk protein and concentrated fat.

Since we have already discussed the basic unfavorable qualities of cow dairy, it should be even more so concerning to note that it takes almost ten pounds of milk to make one pound of cheese. This means that the unfavorable qualities of milk, especially in a cheese derived from cow's milk, are much more concentrated and acidifying.

In addition to the higher-fat content, the casein found in cow dairy is what makes the concentrated version of cow cheeses highly congesting and slow to digest. The pasteurization of cheese is designed to increase shelf-stability and also to kill off potential pathogens for "safe" consumption.

Cheese has a low pH. Cheeses, especially pasteurized cow cheeses, are highly acidifying and have a very low pH.

Cheese is pasteurized. In addition to killing off potential pathogens, the pasteurization process also destroys and diminishes many of the raw nutrients that would otherwise be found in the cheeses, particularly the beneficial food-digesting enzymes needed to break down the concentrated fat and protein.

Young, softer cheese is more susceptible to unwanted bacteria than aged, hard cheese. In the United States, raw cheeses are not permitted for commercial sale unless the cheese has been aged at least 60 days. As a cheese ages, it no longer holds the bacterial risks associated with young cheeses, and thus unpasteurized, or raw cheeses, from a reputable and safe source, are safer for consumption. Therefore, if you wish to enjoy cheese, aged, unpasteurized cheese is preferable.

Aged cheese is easier to digest. Additionally, with age, lactase, the naturally occurring enzyme in cheese, will digest the milk sugar, lactose. Aged cheese will contain virtually no lactose, making it easier to digest.

Cheese contains mold spores. All cheeses contain mold spores and are therefore highly susceptible to mold, causing allergies and worsening conditions associated with bad bacteria imbalances and toxic yeasts like candida. As stated in the previous chapter, candida feeds off of mold-containing foods.

Not all cheeses are created equally. "Cheese foods," like the standard "American cheese" and many presliced cheeses, are highly processed and toxic to the body. With so many added fillers, salts, and flavor enhancers, the food is difficult for the body to break down and digest completely. Incomplete digestion clogs our intestinal piping system and digestive tract, and indirectly affects the skin.

Cheese Alternatives

I do suggest forgoing, or significantly reducing all cheeses for the most radiant complexion, and substituting in nutritional yeast for a "cheesy" flavor. However, if you feel you must eat a little cheese, raw sheep's milk and raw goat's milk cheeses still contain enzymes that will help aid in digestion and have significantly less casein than cow's milk. A goat cheese contains more protein and slightly less fat than a sheep cheese. Sheep cheese is generally a bit saltier and higher in fat. Depending on the individual, I find that different clients may prefer one to the other, as far as taste preference, but also digestion. If you cannot find raw cheeses, a pasteurized goat or sheep cheese is still superior to consuming a raw cow's milk cheese. I do not suggest using soy, rice, or other processed "vegan" cheeses as a replacement for all animal product cheeses. In many cases, these "cheeses" can be even more processed and acidifying than a raw, unpasteurized goat or sheep cheese.

For a nondairy alternative, nutritional yeast looks like yellow flakes and can be found in many specialty health stores, including Whole Foods Market. Nutritional yeast is inactive, nonliving yeast. Though it is not considered toxic in nature, depending on how it is stored (sometimes in bulk) and also processed, it can become contaminated with mold (as can many spices and seasonings). For those following a strict candida-free diet, I do not recommend nutritional yeast as a staple item. It can be, however, a highly beneficial and satisfying seasoning for those transitioning away from dairy or vegan cheeses. At times I use it when I am looking for a cheesy flavor on salads or vegetable dishes.

SOY

Remove soy products from your diet. Soy is a highly processed plant food that has a strong likelihood for increasing inflammation and causing a hefty amount of digestive upset. There are a number of reasons to avoid soy.

The soy products found on our supermarket shelves are rarely in their raw or natural form. So even if soybeans *were* a "healthy" source of protein, the soy products commonly seen are treated and processed. In order to produce products like soy milk, the soy is heated to extremely high temperatures, and then laced with preservatives, stabilizers, and sweeteners.

Soybeans contain enzyme inhibitors. Enzyme inhibitors keep the enzymes needed for protein digestion from working properly. Soybeans are a source of protein, yet they contain a substance that does not let the body break down this protein. This causes stress on the body leading to bloat, indigestion, and constipation, among other negative reactions. These factors affect the skin.

Soy is high in phytic acid. Phytates, like those found in grains, inhibit the body's absorption of calcium, magnesium, iron, and zinc.

Unless a soy product is labeled as organic, it is most likely genetically modified and treated with herbicides. When something is genetically modified, it means that its original chemical makeup is altered so that it can resist toxic fertilizers—thus farmers can grow more and more low-quality and less expensive soy. Downsides? Fertilizers are ingested. GMO foods are not natural and should be avoided.

Soy is grown monoculturally. The agricultural practice of growing soy, also common to mainstream staple foods such as corn and wheat, is called "monoculture." The idea of using this farming practice is to grow a single crop in the same area, year after year. The issue? As Mark Bittman writes in *Food Matters*, "Monoculture doesn't return nutrients to the soil, so it can't be effective without the chemical fertilizers." This means that produce grown in these soils requires more poison be used on the food that will potentially end up on our plates and in our bodies. Unfortunately, these fertilizers are not just a topical nuisance, but are absorbed into the plants themselves.

Soy has the ability to alter hormonal levels. Soy contains phytoestrogens. These compounds mimic human estrogens and have the ability to disrupt the normal functioning of the system of glands, which secrete these hormones directly into the bloodstream (otherwise known as the endocrine system). Estrogens then build up in the blood. While they are slow to initiate noticeable disruption, the results of hormonal changes are much more prolonged.

Soy products are highly processed. Due to the vast amount of processing that goes into producing soy products, it is a fairly common "allergen" whether recognized or not. Similar to cow's milk, soy products are considered quite congesting and thus not only slow digestion but also stimulate mucus production.

The elimination of soy beverages and food products from the diet will improve skin's appearance by improving digestion, eliminating the risk for hormonal imbalances, and reducing the risk of digesting chemical fertilizers. Additionally, other "allergies" may significantly dissipate as a result.

Soy Alternatives

Unless you're using minimal amounts of organic tofu or edamame to transition away from a traditional Western diet of fast and processed food (or a diet heavy in animal meats), it is recommended that soy be completely removed from the diet while you're on the Clear Skin Detox plan.

For soy milk alternatives, I recommend almond, coconut, or hazelnut milks (preferably unsweetened, not just "sugar-free"). If needed, an alcohol-free stevia product, such as NuStevia, can be used. It is not advisable to use rice milk as an alternative due to excessive sugars in rice, which spike insulin levels.

MEAT

If red meat and poultry is to be consumed at all, it should be of the best quality, and consumed minimally. The quality of meat is largely dependent on the diet of the animal and its living quarters. The terms, "grass-fed," "free-range," "wild," and "local" are all indicators of quality. A grain-free, grass-fed diet is the preferred meal plan for animals. You also want to look for meat that is both hormone- and antibiotic-free. However, these are reasons to avoid meat.

Animals raised for consumption are generally treated poorly. In order to mass-produce meat inexpensively, animals are raised in overpopulated and often unclean and horrific environments. These animals are treated with an abundance of antibiotics to avoid the spread of disease and bacteria (an inevitable result from their living conditions). Antibiotics are transferred from animal, to meat, to plate, to bloodstream. The quality of life and the food that factory-farmed animals receive is nothing short of disturbing and detrimental to the quality of meat we purchase. For more information on food industry practices, please check out the following documentaries, because what you don't know *will* hurt you: *Food, Inc.*, *Super Size Me,* and *Forks Over Knives.*

Animal feed is of poor quality, yielding poor-quality meat. In addition to their food's quality, animals were not intended to digest the types of food given to sustain them for slaughter. Cows for instance, would naturally choose to graze on grass and not leftover gruel, or at best, cheap soy and corn. The phrase "We are what we eat" reigns true for animals also. Our health is only as good as the foods it receives as nourishment, and the quality of meat is only as good as the foods used to feed it. Even animals raised on organic feed are not ideal. This generally just means that the animals are being fed organic soy and corn meal, which are, once again, not intended for their consumption.

Animal products are generally dyed. In order to appeal to the eye, animal products (beef, poultry, and fish included) are colored with dyes to appear fresher, more vibrant, and more aesthetically appealing.

The human digestive system was not intended for the regular consumption of meat. A carnivorous animal for instance—say, a cheetah—has a digestive tract roughly 3 feet long. Meat is able to travel readily through the digestive system of the animal, which leaves very little time for decay. In contrast, the human digestive tract is about 25 feet long, meaning meat spends much longer in the body. When meat sits, it decays, putrefies, and smells rancid. This occurs from within the body as well. The long human digestive tract is slow to eliminate animal products, thus encouraging decay from within and an old, ruddy, imperfect complexion.

Carnivorous animals feast on meat that is caught fresh and consumed raw. Animals (with a few exceptions, such as vultures) in the wild will not touch meat that is left too long. The vast majority of mainstream meats go through a series of processes to ensure less risk of bacteria and contamination. While this may ensure a decrease in bacteria, it is just another step away from being considered "fresh."

Animals do not feast on meat daily. The body needs time to recover and rest. Humans have the "luxury" to consume meat and other animal products at every meal, and then some, inhibiting the body from being able to rest properly.

Animal products have a high pH. They are acidic, lowering the body's opportunity for balance.

Skin is best nourished with a diet rich in raw, living plant foods. Plant foods receive most of their nourishment from the sun, therefore providing the body with vitamins, minerals, and essential amino acids. For the most perfect complexion, consumption of meat should be greatly reduced and then eliminated, and then should only be consumed with green vegetables to aid in digestion and decrease acidity.

Remember, tofu and other processed soy products do not serve as good alternatives to meat products when trying to improve digestion and skin health.

When I work with a client who is consuming a high percentage of animal products, the first step we take is to reduce their intake of meat and always serve it with green vegetables, and to eliminate having grains at the same meal. This is preferred to the immediate replacement with soy, processed meat alternatives, or refined grains (like vegan pizza, crackers, and breads). Land animals are significantly more acid-forming than sea animals. The common rule of thumb I give with my clients is that the harder something is to chew usually indicates that it is also more challenging to digest. Red meat can be considerably more acid-forming than a locally raised or organic chicken. However, there are so many factors that contribute to the health and quality of an animal in this day and age that it can be challenging to immediately pinpoint one as less toxic than another. The consumption of any animal, especially a land animal fed an unnatural diet in an unnatural environment will be detrimental to the kidneys, liver, heart, and the skin. A lean meat is not an indicator of health.

Meat Alternatives

Eggs can be a beneficial alternative to those consuming an animal-based diet. Though still acid-forming, local, free-range, and organic eggs can be a satisfying replacement for poultry and red meat.

Enjoy the whole egg, not just the egg white. Egg whites contain albumin, a protein that can be just as slow to digest as the concentrated protein found in milk. The egg yolk contains beneficial vitamins and minerals that are not found in the white of the egg.

In most cases, eggs are less acid-forming and faster to digest than red meat and poultry. The easiest form of egg to digest is a hard-boiled egg. When the egg whites are fried, they become a gluey substance that is harmful to the kidneys and liver, and more challenging to digest.

Leave eggs for the end of the day. If you like to eat omelets, enjoy them for dinner instead of at breakfast. This will help ensure your body has the energy it needs to get through your day, rather than forcing it to focus on digestion. To enhance digestion, eat eggs on a bed of raw greens, like spinach or romaine, and with the addition of a variety of vegetables. Spinach, bell peppers, onions, and fresh herbs not only add satisfying flavor, but also provide the body with filling fibers and enzymes that will help to digest and then sweep out the meal. I recommend serving eggs with a side of lightly steamed broccoli, and/or zucchini. Eat eggs separate from grains and other animal products for enhanced digestion, and radiant skin. You may add a sprinkle of raw goat or sheep cheese for additional flavor.

SEAFOOD

Due to its promising anti-inflammatory response in the body, the health world became obsessed with omega-3 fatty acids. Because of this, fish oil supplements and seafood, especially cuts of salmon, became overnight celebrities.

We have all experienced the internal stressor, inflammation, when we get hurt. At the injured site, the body will become hot, swollen, and flushed pink. These are indicators that the immune system is working and sending out its army of white blood cells and proteins to protect against potential invaders and infection. In this instance, inflammation is a good thing.

When inflammation is prolonged, it creates unwanted stressors on the body, and leaks continuous pro-inflammatory reactions on the body. Low-level inflammation can lead to chronic inflammatory diseases such as various cancers, heart disease, asthma, osteoarthritis, kidney problems, and Alzheimer's. Inflammation also appears on the skin, and can rapidly increase aging, diminishing a youthful, glowing complexion. Chronic inflammation not only makes the complexion appear ruddy and uneven, but also creates digestive issues, fuels candida, speeds aging and premature wrinkles, and becomes a catalyst for unwanted skin disorders such as psoriasis and acne.

Our body responds to the foods we eat by either creating an inflammatory effect (pro-aging) or an anti-inflammatory effect (anti-aging) in the body. Naturally occurring omega-3 fatty acids are considered anti-inflammatory, whereas naturally occurring omega-6 fatty acids are considered inflammatory. The typical Western diet is heavy on foods that contain the inflammatory fatty acid. These include meats, dairy products, potatoes, vegetable oils, corn, rice, processed foods, and most grains, especially refined grains. Worst are the meats and dairy products derived from animals that are fed diets high in omega-6s (grain-fed animals). This is true of seafood also.

Although fish is the more digestible and less acid-forming alternative to poultry and meat, farmed-raised fish, particularly salmon, which is often touted for its healthy skin benefits, does not support superior health or a radiant complexion.

Salmon can be highly inflammatory. While wild salmon has shown to have an anti-inflammatory effect on the body, farm-raised salmon have shown to be highly inflammatory. Farm-raised salmon are fed cereal grains, soy, and corn (and sometimes poultry litter and hydrolyzed chicken feathers), whereas wild salmon enjoy a natural diet rich in algae and shrimp.

Farmed fish are crammed into crowded pens, and showered with antibiotics and pesticides. There is nothing natural about this captivity.

All fish are not created equal. Bottom-dwellers, like shrimp and lobster eat garbage off the ocean floor and filter this garbage throughout their bodies. They are not beautifying. This is not far-fetched, considering that they are also a common allergen in both adults and humans.

Many fish contain mercury. Certain fish, like swordfish, shark, ahi, and big-eye tuna, tilefish, orange roughy, mackerel, and marlin are considered high in mercury. Mercury is a contaminant that affects the nervous system and brain development.

Healthier Fish and Sea "Food" Alternatives

Though I do not feel that eating fish is necessarily beautifying or beneficial, you will not catch me insisting my clients stop eating fish altogether. While certain seafood, like wild-caught salmon, can be a good source of omega-3s, it takes more than adding in a piece of fish to reduce and reverse inflammation.

Not all fish are high in mercury. Fish that are generally considered low in mercury are Alaskan cod, wild salmon, snapper, sea trout, skipjack tuna, bass, halibut, and mahi mahi.

Sashimi is fine in moderation. Sushi, which is the combination of rice, a sticky grain, and fish, an animal product, does not combine well for superior digestion and beautiful skin. When dining out, I recommend enjoying raw or cooked seafood with an abundance of greens and vegetables, and not consuming it with edamame, a soybean and legume, or grains.

Eat more sea veggies. A high-protein and delicious way to enjoy the benefits of the sea is to add sea vegetables like nori and dulse to recipes. I personally love to recommend that my clients use nori sheets as tortillas and wrap up salads in them like a burrito or sandwich. Dulse can be a unique way to dress up a salad with mineral-rich and salty flavor. Try to avoid seaweed salads. While they can be delicious and flavorful, they are often not made fresh and sit in an abundance of soy and sesame oils.

PEANUT BUTTER

Peanuts are quite misleading in the sense that they are not nuts, but rather legumes. They are a root cause for weight gain and other common skin concerns, such as acne, and topical disorders like eczema and itchy rashes. All peanut products should be removed from the diet for the best immediate results and a clear complexion. Here are a few other reasons to avoid peanut products and peanut oils.

Peanuts are some of the most difficult-to-digest legumes. Slow digestion leads to accumulation and excess waste and weight in the body, becoming the perfect breeding ground for organisms that weaken immunity and damage the skin.

Stored peanuts easily become moldy. This mold is none other than aflatoxin—a *toxic* mold that is thought to be a carcinogen (cancer-causing). Candida albicans, toxic yeasts contributing to common skin disorders like acne and aging, feeds off of mold. Peanuts can help this toxic organism rapidly reproduce and colonize in the body.

A variety of health stores offer freshly ground peanut butters. These peanut butters can be made, in seconds, right before your eyes, sans additives. The concern is that unless thoroughly cleansed daily, these machines may be at even more of a risk for being contaminated with mold.

Peanut butter has additives. Most manufactured and jarred peanut butters not only contain the high fat content of the peanut alone, but are also loaded up on hydrogenated oils, sugar, salt, and dextrose (in addition to other additives). This makes the peanut spread even more indigestible.

Peanuts are highly acid-forming.

Peanuts are addicting. Addiction is a sign of toxicity.

Peanut Butter Alternatives

Raw almond butter, raw tahini (freshly ground sesame seeds), and even sunbutter (roasted sunflower seed spread), can be less acid-forming than peanut butter and are generally easier to digest. Raw nuts and seeds are always preferred to roasted. Heating delicate fats can cause the food to become rancid and therefore damaging to the skin and cells.

For radiant skin, dense fats with a high concentration of protein, like nuts and seeds, should not be consumed with meats or grains. For ideal digestion and a beautiful complexion, use with raw vegetables or in salad dressings in place of oils. Another good transition food and a better substitute for peanut butter is oil-free hummus. Though beans and legumes are generally gas-forming, and not an ideal source of beauty food, they are an inexpensive form of protein, and can be an excellent way to transition away from traditional dips and condiments like peanut butter.

SUGAR

Sugar has been shown to be just as addictive as "stimulant drugs" like cocaine. Just as sugar residue contributes to the rotting of the teeth, it is destructive internally as well. Although it is unrealistic to assume we can remove all sugar from the diet, all sugar, even the sugar found in whole fruit, should be eaten in moderation. Processed sugars, like high-fructose corn syrup, and most sugar substitutes, like sucrose and aspartame, should be eliminated. Other foods that should be avoided include agave nectar, as well as cooked foods that are too quickly converted into sugar in the body without also supplying additional nutrients and food enzymes. These include white potatoes, rice, and refined grains. Other reasons to avoid and limit sugar:

Sugar is acidic. After sugar is metabolized, it leaves behind an acid ash, or residue, that lowers the body's pH. This invites the types of disease and bacteria that wreak havoc on the skin.

Sugar feeds bacteria. As sugar ferments, it actually feeds the bacteria, candida, viruses, and parasites, extending their life and worsening the condition of the skin.

Sugar substitutes are likely to be even more acid-forming than processed sugars. Regardless of whether they "start out as sugar," the majority of sugar substitutes are so highly processed, that the body is unable to recognize and break them down to use for energy. Sucralose, for instance, is a fancy name for a sugar molecule whose "natural" chemical structure has been altered by replacing hydroxyl groups with chlorine atoms. This causes the body not to recognize it as sugar, but it does not mean it is not stored elsewhere. There is absolutely nothing natural or beautifying about this overused and abused sweetener.

Sugar hides in just about everything we consume, from soda pops and desserts to more unsuspecting items like ketchup, dressings, and packaged snacks and crackers. Processed starches, like most "traditional" rice (white and brown), breads, packaged snacks, and crackers are converted to sugar in the body. They can be even bigger offenders because they are void of natural nutrients *and* take much longer to digest.

Alternatives to Sugar and Sugar Alternatives

Stevia is an herb known for its almost potent sweetness. Although it has now been mass-produced, and often in forms that are not always favorable, it is one of the best sweeteners on the market today. Avoid the white powdered variety, as it generally contains dextrose, a simple sugar, and maltodextrin, a digestible carbohydrate made from cornstarch. Although these additives are not particularly harmful, if alcohol-free liquid forms are available to you, this is the better way to go. Additionally, erythritol and xylitol can be used in moderation as less-offensive sweeteners than their synthetic and artificial counterparts, aspartame, saccharin, and sucralose.

Remember, candida does not discriminate. It loves sugar. If you are not overly concerned with candida, raw, local honey can be a wonderful sweetener in moderation. I like to add 1 tablespoon of raw honey to 1½ cups hot water with fresh squeezed lemon in the morning. I also will use grade B maple syrup in special recipes, especially when entertaining and around the holidays. Grade B maple syrup is significantly less processed and ideally contains more nutrients than common grade A maple syrup. Medjool dates also can serve as a sweetener in desserts and dressings, for those not concerned with candida or bacterial imbalance.

CAFFEINE AND STIMULANTS

Caffeine is a stimulant and affects the body's normal functioning. Similar to the stimulant found in chocolate (theobromine), caffeine is responsible for temporarily increasing heart rate, raising blood pressure, relaxing the smooth muscles on the bronchi in the lungs, opening airways, and increasing mental clarity. Because of these factors, it is also considered an aphrodisiac. However, along with these seemingly positive attributes is a negative consequence. Therefore there are a number of reasons to avoid and limit caffeine and stimulants.

Caffeine is acidic. Natural sources of caffeine, like coffee, tea, and chocolate, can be addictive substances that are acid-forming and lower the body's pH. When consumed in excess, especially in addition to a Westernized diet, caffeine can exacerbate common skin conditions like acne and rosacea.

Caffeine is a diuretic. All caffeine works as a diuretic and can deplete the body of water and dehydrate the skin. Dry skin signifies imbalance and is often a result of diet, lifestyle, and environmental factors like cold temperatures or too much sun. Dryness can make skin appear rough, flaky, red, itchy, and cracked.

Without sufficient hydration, the skin loses its elasticity and can lead to fine lines and wrinkles, especially around the eyes, mouth, and forehead.

Dehydration also disrupts and slows blood circulation. With poor circulation there is a delay in the body's ability to rid itself of toxins. Toxic overload can lead to serious health complications in addition to imperfect skin.

Caffeine increases stress. Caffeine can elevate the hormone cortisol, which can increase stress levels and aggravate and stress the adrenal glands. The adrenal glands are responsible for producing the stress hormones adrenaline and cortisol in response to our busy and hectic lives. When the body is under chronic and constant "stress," it loses its ability to respond appropriately and struggles to maintain balance. Adrenal fatigue can cause a number of unwanted side effects, including anxiety, mood swings, hormonal imbalances, cravings, exhaustion, and sleeplessness, to name just a few. It also causes us to *look* exhausted, and it contributes to dark under-eye circles, wrinkles, increased aging, and acne.

Caffeine is addictive.

Caffeine causes inflammation. While coffee may help some individuals keep regular, it also aggravates and creates inflammation for the intestinal walls. This can lead to allergies, including blemishes that appear as an indirect result of inflamed intestinal tissue.

When the skin is already suffering and the body is out of balance, caffeinated beverages, although commonly touted for their antioxidants, do not supply significant enough nutrients to offset this balance. In fact, they may also be removing nutrients without giving back to the community. I call them "takers." They are not givers.

If you are drinking coffee or green tea for increased energy, you will soon find all caffeine, for the sake of energy and mental clarity, is unnecessary. That being said, I do not rule out coffee or cocoa from a client's diet, especially when there are bigger fish to fry. Without fiber, a natural beverage like coffee or green tea requires virtually no digestion. So although acid-forming and a cause of inflammation, it does not require the same burdensome affect that processed, dairy, and meat products do for the body. I ask that clients limit their intake to one cup, and at most, two cups of coffee, or homemade Hot Cacao (page 184) a day, and switch to herbal teas and lemon water. I also realize that for many, coffee can be a ritual experience. I certainly love the aromas of freshly ground coffee beans. If you are looking for a quick turnaround in your skin, I would not recommend coffee as your source of energy or antioxidants, or for regularity. However, I would also not put it at the top of your list to completely eliminate from the get-go.

Alternatives to Caffeine and Stimulants

What you really want in your diet is something that keeps on giving. In other words, you want a source of nourishment that enriches your every cell with enzymes, raw vitamins, minerals, and natural sugars and literally flushes the body with alkalinity, instead of merely pulling nutrients from the body as it acidifies.

While beverages containing caffeine can be detrimental to the skin, others can be highly detoxifying, hydrating, alkalizing, and can actually work to restore cell regeneration while reversing aging, and completely eliminating acne and other unwanted skin disorders. This life-enhancing, skin-beautifying beverage I speak of is raw, freshly pressed fruit and vegetable juice.

Because the body absorbs nutrients through the human tissue of the intestines, the most nourishing thing one can do for the body is to infuse it with freshly pressed vegetable juice before breakfast and after drinking pure water. When consumed on an empty stomach, freshly pressed, unpasteurized vegetable juice is the equivalent to taking several "shots" of raw vitamins, minerals, and essential "energy-boosting" plant sugars.

Juicing, not to be confused with blending (or smoothies), is a process that removes the indigestible fibers from fruits and vegetables. What remains of the living plant is the water, vegetable glucose (sugar), enzymes, and living nutrients (vitamins and minerals). Without requiring digestion, freshly pressed juice is able to quickly provide the most abundant source of alkaline nutrients to the body. Although fiber is essential, juicing greens, root vegetables, and fruits gives the body access to nutrients it would be unrealistic for it to consume, let alone digest, otherwise.

For instance, you can drink and digest the nutrient equivalent of five pounds of carrots juiced much more readily than the same amount in the blended form of a soup or smoothie.

The enzymes in juice also loosen impacted waste from the intestines and colon, aiding the body in elimination, greatly improving digestion, and healing the colon from the inside out. The juice of certain root vegetables, like beets, carrots, and ginger, can actually stimulate our peristalsis muscle and transport and eliminate skin-damaging wastes out of the body. Peristalsis is the contraction and relaxation of the digestive system. The intestines rely on peristaltic movement to move waste from the small intestine to the large intestine for elimination.

BENEFITS OF JUICING AND GREEN SMOOTHIES

Imagine consuming six pounds of raw vegetables in one day. Now imagine consuming a highly concentrated beverage with the equivalent of those vegetables in *one* 16-ounce juice. Freshly pressed and unpasteurized juice is absolutely incredible because it virtually bypasses digestion in the stomach, and it infuses the body with a highly alkaline and nutrient-dense beverage that is absorbed straight into the bloodstream.

A smoothie can be a nutrient-dense food that is rich in fiber, and more easily digested than the ingredients in their whole form. Food that requires more time to digest, or is more challenging to break down in the stomach, steals energy from the body. The goal of the stomach is to break down a meal completely and properly before it continues on to the small intestine. During the blending process, ingredients are "pulverized." This process is the equivalent of us chewing our food the correct amount of times before swallowing—we can call this "pre-digesting." Once food reaches the small intestine, nutrient absorption can occur. A meal must be completely and properly broken down in order for the small intestine to fully benefit from the food's nutrients.

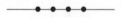

GRAINS

Whole grains are often highly regarded since they are high sources of fiber. However, misleading is the mass marketing of "high-fiber" foods, which strip the whole food of its nutrients, leaving only the indigestible fiber left for consumption. Foods labeled as being a "good source of fiber" or "containing whole grains" or "made with whole grains," can be deceptive and fool us into thinking that a product is beneficial. In fact, the majority of these foods have little to no nutritional value, and so adding fiber can make the product seem more appealing and temporarily filling. Processed and refined grains and flours have also been stripped of any redeeming qualities and can slow digestion, create and worsen inflammation, and serve only to fill a belly while feeding bacteria and toxic yeasts like candida.

Gluten, a protein found in wheat, is highly inflammatory. Not only is it linked to digestive issues, irritable bowel syndrome, and the like, but it can also contribute to a variety of skin issues and complications, like cystic acne, which appears as large and inflamed raised bumps, that can ooze with pus. In addition to creating intestinal irritation and sensitivity, gluten and refined grains can create puncture wounds in the intestinal lining, and can cause our bodies to leak large proteins, waste, and undigested foods into the bloodstream. This increased permeability, known as Leaky Gut Syndrome, can cause us to become highly sensitive and develop allergies to other foods, even foods otherwise deemed healthy.

Alternatives to Grain

Fiber is a necessity in any diet. In addition to beneficial enzymes, it cleanses the colon, acting like an "intestinal" broom. However, the type of fiber we choose is instrumental in the appearance of the skin.

"Fiber" is the simple term used to describe the protective cell wall, or plant cellulose, that protects and is a part of every plant. Because we cannot digest the greater majority of plant cellulose, or fiber, the bulk of it can help to sweep out skin-damaging toxins.

It is easy to get enough fiber when we are eating a whole-food, plant-based diet. Fiber can effortlessly be consumed in abundance through the daily intake of vegetables.

To be most effective in its sweeping, and to quickly exit the digestive tract, fiber should be consumed in its whole form. This simply means that the fiber found in an apple, or lightly steamed broccoli, is much more readily digested and cleansing than is the fiber found in overcooked, processed, and mass-marketed "high-fiber" cereals, grains, foods, and supplements. In fact, the natural plant waters found in fresh vegetables aid in their "clean up," and quicker release, hydrating the internal organs instead of dehydrating and depleting them of minerals.

It is OK and even beneficial to lightly cook vegetables too. Vegetables with a high-fiber profile generally have a smaller water-to-fiber ratio. This can mean they will be harder to digest, and thus the light steaming of these fibrous vegetables (specifically broccoli, Brussels sprouts, cauliflower, and cabbage) tenderizes the fibrous solids and makes digestion easier and cleansing. Lightly steaming will help to keep enzymes intact, whereas overcooking will destroy all digestive-enhancing food enzymes.

Though whole fruits also contain fiber, for clearer and more radiant skin, it is best to focus the majority of fiber intake on alkalizing greens and vegetables, which are much lower in sugar and higher in protein. Fruit is a very clean food, high in water and sugar. If the body is too acidic, or housing sugar-feasting bacteria and yeasts like candida, the fruit sugars do little to cleanse and may only cause more discomfort and fermentation. Until the body is in better balance, it is best to limit fruit intake. We will discuss fruit in further detail in the next few chapters.

The General Grocery Shopping List (page 200) is designed to help you navigate your grocery store based on your dietary preferences and current lifestyle. It will help you better understand what your alternatives are when looking to supplement your diet with healthier options. Allowing yourself to transition, rather than jump right into a new nutrition plan "cold turkey," can reduce feelings of restriction and will help you to build healthy habits you will love!

CHAPTER 3

Everyday Foods for Beautiful Skin

Don't be fooled into thinking you have to purchase oddly named, exotic foods to experience the benefits of superior well-being. The Big Food and supplement industries love to capitalize on our society's desire for a quick fix or a magic pill. However, when we better understand how every substance that enters the body has some sort of effect on the entire system, we are better able to understand the value and role each piece of food can play and how they work together.

You will not need a dictionary to decipher the following foods. Many of these items are readily available at your local grocer, if not larger specialty markets, health stores, Asian markets, and farmer's markets. While there are many other foods that can be added to this list, I chose superfoods that almost everyone will be able to integrate into their diet.

APPLES (ORGANIC)

The expression "An apple a day keeps the doctor away" does have some merit. Apples can pack in a small share of nutrients in each bite. They contain small amounts of free radical–fighting vitamin

A and modest amounts of vitamin C, a precursor to collagen production and an antioxidant. Apples are a good source of vitamin K and offer a small amount of vitamin E, as well as a smattering of some of the B vitamins. Apples contain a healthy dose of calcium, magnesium, and, most notably, potassium. They also contain apple pectin, a phytonutrient that has been recognized for its powerful detoxifying and cleansing properties.

Biting into an apple can help scrub away debris from the teeth. In addition, depending on the soil in which they are grown, apples can be a good source of fluoride. Fluoride can be found readily in plant foods. It is also naturally available in the ocean. Due to its natural ability to support strong teeth and bones, fluoride has long since been added to our water sources and dental care products. This is a hotly debated topic, as it is considered poisonous in the degrees to which we are drinking it outside of our diet. You don't need to be concerned about supplementing your diet with fluoride-fortified products when the better solution is to choose calcium-rich foods and limit sugary foods that not only cause tooth decay, but rapid aging, acne, and skin disorders.

As with all fruit, apples should only be consumed on an empty stomach. Since apples can stimulate activity in the small intestine, if you're experiencing diarrhea from apple consumption, it may have something to do with an existing blockage of waste and inflammation in the intestines that the food is addressing. Apples are also an excellent source of fiber.

It is wise to avoid apples unless you can budget for organic. It has been cited that over 30 different types of pesticides have been detected on nonorganic apples. If the food you are eating can wipe out a whole colony of bugs, it is probably best to leave them out of your diet.

ARUGULA

Arugula is a highly alkaline and anti-inflammatory plant, rich in folate, antioxidant vitamins A and C as well as vitamin K. Vitamin K promotes strong bones and healthy blood circulation, and helps the bones to better absorb calcium. Arugula's peppery leaves are cleansing and promote beauty from within with its superior concentration of free radical–fighting antioxidants that not only help to ward off signs of aging, but also encourage cell reproduction, collagen support, and strengthen the optic and immune systems.

Arugula is also a good source of calcium and magnesium, which are necessary for strength, detoxification, and stress management, as well as iron absorption, which is required to oxygenate the various systems of the body.

ASPARAGUS

Asparagus is a good source of immune-boosting vitamin C as well as age-defying antioxidant vitamin A.

Asparagus is low in calories and sodium, but an excellent source of potassium and water, making it hydrating, while it is also beneficial as a diuretic, helping to alleviate the body of excess water.

Like arugula, asparagus is a great source of vitamin K, a fat-soluble vitamin that supports the body in the absorption of calcium, and is also rich in silicon, a mineral found in human nails, connective tissue, cartilage, and bones, giving them firmness and strength.

Dr. Norman W. Walker, a pioneer in holistic health, digestion and medicine, considered asparagus to be a highly cleansing vegetable, supportive of the kidneys and bladder in their detoxification, for which the skin serves as a backup organ. This means that eating asparagus helps cleanse those primary detox organs, leaving the skin clearer.

AVOCADOS

Avocados are a unique fruit. At roughly 300 calories, 30 grams of fat, and 5 grams of protein, an avocado is highly concentrated in nutrients, calories, and fat and physically denser than most fruit, with the exception of bananas.

Avocados are one of the highest-quality sources of fat we can put into the body. Unfortunately, it is typically these high calorie and fat contents that have us avoiding and replacing the avocado with lesser-quality oils and fat-free alternatives, when in fact a moderate amount of fat, about half an avocado a day, is essential for a radiant complexion. Additionally, avocados are a package deal, containing the fat-digesting enzyme lipase, which actually helps to break down and digest the fat itself for increased digestion, metabolism, and overall support.

Avocados are also a great source of magnesium. Magnesium is an alkaline mineral required by every system and function in the body, integral to the body's natural detoxification process, aiding in the relaxation of the intestines, and thus also the easy elimination of waste.

Avocados are a good source of potassium, an electrolyte that helps the body to regulate and maintain water, as well as iron and manganese—which support healthy circulation and regulate body temperature.

Although technically a fruit, their uncharacteristic consistency and high fat content is slower to digest than most fruit. When properly combined with other foods, such as sweet potatoes, winter squashes, greens, and both starchy (ex: peas, cooked carrots, and corn) and low starch vegetables (ex: zucchini, summer squash, broccoli), avocados are easily broken down by the body and provide immune-strengthening support with vitamin C, and antiaging, free radical–fighting antioxidants vitamins A and E. For detoxification and enhanced digestion that promotes healthy skin, avocados combine nicely with starches. They can also be combined with bananas, dried fruit, and young Thai coconuts, but never animal proteins, nuts, or seeds.

BASIL AND MINT

Often sprinkled into pasta dishes, or made into pesto, basil and mint are beneficial relatives and promote clear, even skin from the inside out. In addition to basil's rock star vitamin and mineral content, most notably vitamins K and A, iron, calcium, and magnesium, fresh basil leaves are considered to have valuable anti-inflammatory, antibacterial, and antifungal properties.

Free radical–fighting antioxidants combat aging by preserving the cells from damage. Iron oxygenates the blood and provides healthy circulation to the skin. Alkaline minerals promote a balanced pH.

Easy to add into juices, smoothies, salads, and vegetable marinades, fresh basil and mint are more than just garnishes.

BEETS

Beets are a beauty food. Packed with nutrients necessary for a youthful, glowing complexion, beets not only offer a sufficient amount of naturally occurring vitamins and minerals, but also support a healthy digestive system. Like most fresh produce, beets are alkaline and can contribute to finding balance in the body, but they are also considered anti-inflammatory and help to ease inflammation.

Naturally high in fiber and an excellent source of food enzymes, beets are highly cleansing, helping to naturally stimulate digestion. They are also a great source of magnesium, considered Mother Nature's "relaxant" and stress aid. This alkaline mineral relaxes the skeletal and smooth muscles of the body, including the intestines.

Stressors and other variables cause these muscles to contract, making it more challenging for the body to get rid of toxins. A relaxed digestive tract allows the body to pass waste more easily, thus reducing the buildup of unwanted substances that burden the organs and taint the bloodstream. Beets are also highly beneficial in managing hormonal imbalances, which contribute to stress and skin problems.

Beets are a good source of betaine, a molecule that aids in the detoxification process by helping to neutralize otherwise poisonous metals and substances, making it exceptional for beautiful skin. This root vegetable can help to correct skin issues by helping to reduce the toxic load on the liver and kidneys that can cause our body to eliminate waste through the skin.

BROCCOLI

When very lightly steamed, broccoli florets are like little fibrous brooms, helping to sweep out toxic wastes from the body, aiding in regular and ongoing detoxification of the intestines.

Broccoli is rich in vitamins A and C, making it a powerhouse of free radical–fighting and age-defying nutrients. It is also a good source of calcium, phosphorus, magnesium, and iron, making it supportive of a strong skeletal structure and aiding the body in the circulation of oxygen throughout.

Broccoli is also an excellent source of folate, needed for proper growth and development of all cells. Folate is used therapeutically to treat issues ranging from acne and eczema to depression and fatigue. This B-complex vitamin is also required for the conversion of amino acids into protein, red cell production, and it plays an important role in the reduction of plaque buildup in the arteries.

Eat your broccoli, but don't overcook it. Cruciferous vegetables, like broccoli, cauliflower, and cabbage, are more easily digested when they are just barely steamed, loosening up their tough plant cellulose. That said, overcooking will deplete vitamins and minerals, especially water-soluble vitamins A and C, as well as food-digesting enzymes.

BURDOCK ROOT

When I first started to study the value of herbs in treating acne and various skin disorders, burdock root was one that I found particularly fascinating.

Burdock root can be found in specialty grocers or in most health food stores in supplement form. It is a unique root that has powerful purifying and diuretic properties. Burdock's cleansing action on the kidneys can help the body to more effectively and efficiently eliminate toxins through urine, instead of leaving them for potential recirculation in the bloodstream. This helps the kidneys to function more optimally and focus their attention on self-regeneration. Burdock root is also thought to fight inflammation and protect against bacteria and fungal imbalances, like candida.

Resembling a dark brown twig, burdock root (also referred to as *gobo*) has a dark brown and gray exterior and a bright white center. It can be juiced, tossed into stir-fry dishes, or baked. It is used topically as well as internally.

CARROTS

Carrots are often noted for their high concentration of vitamin A. This water-soluble antioxidant is instrumental in achieving a youthful complexion, as it works to scavenge free radicals running amok in the body and supports a strong immune system.

Carrots are also a great source of vitamin C, another powerful antioxidant that protects the cells against free radical damage.

Vitamin C is the precursor to collagen formation, which promotes tight, supple skin and is important for adrenal support, helping to combat emotional and physical stress, as well as aiding in muscle and tissue repair.

Additionally, carrots are a good source of calcium, iron, and magnesium, making them ideal for strong bones and healthy posture. Carrots also contain selenium, a trace mineral that is considered important for youth and longevity. Selenium is thought to enhance the properties of vitamin E.

Renowned healer Dr. Norman W. Walker considered fresh-pressed carrot juice, to be "a particularly wonderful cleanser of bile and waste matter coagulated in the liver as a result of years of wrong eating." Bile is the fluid secreted by the liver to help aid in fat digestion. Without it, fat would go undigested, creating a greater burden on the liver. Carrot juices are an excellent natural sweetener to add to green juices in place of fruit. Coupled with potent levels of vitamin A from beta-carotene, carrot juice becomes a phenomenal aid to the liver, kidneys, and therefore, skin.

CELERY

Often considered a "diet food" or a "freebie" in many weight-loss programs, celery is an exceptional source of potassium and sodium, electrolytes that help the body regulate and eliminate excess fluid. Celery is also an excellent source of water and fiber, aiding in the detoxification and elimination of impurities while providing hydration.

The mineral-rich water in celery is highly alkalizing, containing alkaline minerals like calcium and magnesium that help to build strong bones, lower blood pressure, and promote proper cardiovascular function. Often recommended in greater doses to clients who suffer from stress and anxiety, foods that contain higher levels of magnesium are also considered naturally calming by having a soothing effect on the nerves and relaxing the smooth muscles in the body. Increased elimination of waste coupled with the soothing effects of magnesium may help to reverse adrenal fatigue, which can make us appear older around our eyes.

Feeling puffy or suffering from dark under-eye circles? Be sure to include celery in your morning juice.

CILANTRO

Cilantro is the leafy offspring of the highly anti-inflammatory coriander seed, which is often ground and used as a spice.

Containing virtually no calories, fat, or sugar, but a superior source of vitamin A, cilantro leaves are a class act for reversing aging and getting a blemish-free complexion. Cilantro is also a valid source of additional free radical–fighting antioxidants, like vitamins E and C, and a rich source of vitamin K, which is needed for calcium absorption.

Cilantro is a good source of folate, which is required for protein conversion, red blood cell production, and a healthy heart. Therapeutically, folate is used to treat issues of the skin and support a healthy state of mind. Due to its high anti-inflammatory response on the body, and superior levels of antioxidants, cilantro is excellent for treating topical skin disorders, such as eczema and acne, but also works to reverse signs of aging. Additionally, it is used to treat depression and anxiety, most likely due to its high mineral content and alkaline qualities.

Cilantro is also considered to hold antibacterial properties and is thought to bind to heavy metals in the body, disposing of them through proper elimination. Heavy metals can build up in our systems due to the equipment we cook with, including aluminum, as well as through the mercury we ingest with regular seafood consumption.

Cilantro is a good source of fiber, and has healing properties when both the stem and leaves are juiced with additional vegetables or added to a green smoothie. Cilantro leaves can be chopped and added to salads, vegetable dishes, and of course, guacamole, for an additional mineral beauty boost.

COLLARDS

Collards are an excellent source of vitamins A, C, K, and E, and a good source of the minerals calcium, potassium, iron, and zinc. Right up there with kale, collards have among the highest concentration of nutrients per calorie and are very low in calories, making each bite beauty-enhancing.

Highly alkaline, collards have anti-inflammatory properties that promote a radiant and glowing complexion. They are also high in enzymes and fiber, promoting regularity and ongoing detoxification.

The leaves of collards can be used in place of flour or corn tortillas, and used as a naturally gluten-free, free radical–fighting alternative to bread and wraps when making a skin-saving sandwich.

CUCUMBER

The expression "cool as a cucumber" has merit. Cucumbers are recognized as a cooling food, decreasing body temperature with consumption, and they are exceptionally hydrating due to their high water content. Their water is rich in the alkaline nutrients potassium, iron, and magnesium, making them calming to the nervous system and important for healthy circulation and hydrated, glowing skin.

Cucumbers are also a great source of silicon, which is required for collagen formation and supports healthy skin, hair, and nails.

When eating cucumbers in their whole form, partially peel the skin from the cucumber before slicing, creating stripes of skin and cucumber flesh. This can help aid digestion. The skin of the cucumber can be saved and thrown into a green smoothie or juiced, as it too contains beneficial nutrients, supportive of youthful radiance.

DANDELION GREENS

Often considered nuisances, dandelions are those bright yellow pops of color that spring up on your front lawn. Dandelion greens, on the other hand, are the dark, leafy, and jagged greens with warming qualities and medicinal properties.

Supportive of the liver in detoxification, dandelion greens aid in the flow of bile and are thus also helpful in reducing stress placed on the gallbladder. Stimulating to the lymph glands, dandelion greens help to remove impurities quickly through the pores.

Dandelion greens contain a high concentration of vitamin A, which is necessary in fighting free radicals that lead to rapid aging and wrinkles. The greens are also a great source of vitamin D, vitamin C, some of the B vitamins, iron, and calcium, as well as potassium and sodium, minerals that balance and regulate hydration of the cells.

Go easy when adding dandelion greens to the diet, especially when juicing. They are best used as a supplement to a diet of wholesome foods because they are powerful enough to create toxic release. Medicinal greens can be an excellent *addition* to your diet for a perfect complexion, because they help the liver release toxins. When we combine these greens with enhanced digestion, the results are powerful. However, when toxins are not leaving the system through the bowel, toxins can be forced to leave through the skin, temporarily exacerbating topical skin disorders. Dandelion greens are considered a medicinal green because they are highly effective in pulling out stored toxins from human tissue. Using dandelions greens as a cleanser means that we must also be strengthening digestive system and the route of elimination. Try adding dandelion leaves to your juice every other day or finely chopping a leaf into your salad daily.

ENDIVE

Endive is a bitter food, sometimes used in salads or medicinally in juices to help aid in the detoxification of the liver and to enhance digestion. It is also considered a good blood purifier, and is therefore helpful in alleviating stress on the liver, as well as helping to eliminate pathogens that may cause aging, acne, and topical skin problems.

Endive is high in antioxidants, including vitamin E, which is of paramount importance for skin health, age reversal, and the prevention of cell damage. In addition to its high antioxidant profile, it is also a considerable source of iron, which keeps blood oxygenated and skin glowing and radiant.

Thought to reduce inflammation, endive is an alkaline food. It is rich in electrolytes as well as calcium.

FENNEL

Fennel is a very alkaline food. Both the bulb and the stems of the fennel are beneficial. Due to the higher concentration of indigestible fibers in the green stalks, the bulb is more easily digested, and the stalks are best for juicing. Grated, thinly chopped, or diced into salads, the bulb can be an excellent digestive aid, stimulating digestion and helping the body eliminate excess water. The same can be said for fennel stalks, which can also help ease inflammation and digestive discomforts, but their properties are more beneficial when juiced, instead of chewed.

According to Dr. Norman W. Walker, fennel is also beneficial in "loosening up mucous or phlegm conditions." The body produces mucus in a protective attempt to collect unwanted pathogens from entering the bloodstream. With excess inflammation and poor dietary and lifestyle choices, the body produces mucus in excess amounts, slowing digestion and acting as a detriment to the body.

GARLIC

Garlic is considered one of Mother Nature's most potent antibiotic and antifungal plants. Its potent odor comes from sulfur and it has been used for centuries for medicinal reasons, as well as to ward off evil spirits. Sulfur has been shown to promote the elimination of toxins from the blood and lymphatic system and is thought to be effective in killing bacteria.

Unlike the vast majority of prescription medications that can harm the internal harmony of good bacteria in the body, regular consumption of garlic leaves the body's healthy bacteria and yeasts unharmed while destroying and halting the colonization of toxic yeasts and bacteria that can cause adrenal stress, hormonal imbalances, depression, acne, and other topical skin disorders.

Best consumed raw, it becomes spicier the more the plant walls are destroyed, so instead of crushing it, try thinly slicing it on a mandolin.

GINGER

It is quite a misconception that the beverage "ginger ale" is soothing to an upset stomach, with all of the soda's indigestible and gas-producing carbonation, sugar, and additives. The principle behind the idea, however, is not without some truth.

Gingerroot has long been used in dishes and tonics to stimulate a sluggish digestion, improving bile flow, helping to strengthen the intestinal muscles, and improving the rate at which waste matter is eliminated from the body. Gingerroot is highly anti-inflammatory and healing to the intestines, which can be aggravated and torn with continuous inflammatory substances and inefficient elimination of waste matter. Once torn, the intestinal lining can become sensitive to different foods and environmental conditions. These sensitivities can present themselves in different ways, including rashes, rosacea, and acne.

Ginger is easy to incorporate slowly into juices, teas, and stir-fry dishes.

KALE

Like most greens, kale is highly alkalizing. Kale is also considered an excellent anti-inflammatory food source, while many processed foods common to modern diets cause inflammation. Excess inflammation leads to rapid aging and the degeneration of cells, auto-immune problems, arthritis, allergies, and a score of unwanted inflammatory issues that detract from the appearance and comfort of the skin.

A phenomenal source of calcium and plant protein, the nutrients in kale support cellular growth, strength, and a healthy metabolism, while antioxidants, vitamins A and C, help ward off aging and cell degeneration. Vitamin K, a fat-soluble vitamin, works in tandem with calcium, helping the bones to better absorb it. It is also important to healthy blood flow.

Kale also contains iron, a trace element found in hemoglobin. Hemoglobin is the protein in red blood cells necessary for the circulation of oxygen to the cells. Poor circulation can result in inefficient transportation of nutrients to the skin, making it slow to heal. It can also result in under-eye circles, dullness or discoloration, aging, and the buildup of impurities. Iron plays an integral role in our DNA, as well as our energy levels.

A great source of fiber and sulfur, kale is naturally detoxifying, supporting a healthy liver and regular elimination of waste.

LEMONS

Lemons are an excellent source of vitamin C, an essential water-soluble antioxidant that must be obtained through the diet, as the body does not produce it on its own. Aside from its paramount importance in a healthy immune system, vitamin C is the main ingredient required for the production of collagen and is necessary for strong bones, teeth, muscles, and youthful, glowing skin.

This water-soluble vitamin is also considered critical in helping the body to recover and heal from wear and tear. It is therefore important in the age-reversal process and for those looking to heal from skin damage.

Because it is a water-soluble vitamin, vitamin C's potency can be easily lost through cooking and thus is best consumed in its raw and unprocessed form. We can also diminish vitamin C levels through frequent urination, therefore diuretics and drinking alcoholic beverages and stimulants can increase our need for vitamin C.

A food may taste acidic, but when foods are metabolized in the body, they either leave off an alkaline or acid residue in the body. Although they taste acidic, lemons are actually alkaline-forming and promote a healthy pH level within the body. We can easily increase our vitamin C levels just by squeezing fresh lemon juice over green salads, as well as adding it to juices and smoothies.

Lemons are also considered instrumental in aiding in the detoxification of the liver, helping with the break down of fats and production of bile. Lemon juice helps to stimulate gastric juices and aid in digestion. I recommend beginning the day with a mug of hot water with fresh squeezed lemon for an alkaline, digestive-friendly, liver-detoxifying start to your morning.

MÂCHE

Mâche is quite possibly one of my favorite "luxury" greens because its leaves are so fluffy and tender in texture, and so mild and surprisingly nutty in flavor. Like microgreens and sprouts, mâche is a little more challenging to come by and because of its price tag, it can be more cost effective to grow at home than some greens.

Mâche is a phenomenal source of potassium, an important electrolyte required for ideal hydration and elimination of water retention. It is also an excellent source of omega-3 fatty acids. The ratio of omega-3, -6, and -9 is extremely important for age reversal and skin health due to its influence on inflammation in the body. Omega-3 fatty acids have an *anti*-inflammatory response in the body, whereas omega-6 and omega-9 can have an *in*flammatory response in the body. This is important because the majority of foods we consume today have a disproportionately high ratio of omega-6 and -9 fatty acids compared to omega-3s. This is related to the environment in which food is raised, in addition to our dependency on animal products and processed foods.

Like most greens, mâche is highly alkaline, and an excellent source of minerals. It is also a good source of iron, which supports healthy circulation and oxygenation to the skin, as well as protein. Mâche is a good source of antioxidants, like A and C.

MICROGREENS

If you are a greens aficionado, or a frequent health food shopper, you have undoubtedly come in contact with leafy greens labeled "baby," differentiating "baby romaine" from its crisper older sister or "baby kale" from its more robust and cruciferous brother. Foods that are considered "baby," though often more expensive, are less mature versions of greens.

Just as with any living thing, as we age, we grow tougher, and break down. This is also true for mixed greens, which become more fibrous and begin to lose their nutrients as they mature in the fields. When picked prior to maturity, baby greens can have significantly higher levels of nutrients in relatively small amounts. Far more delicate, baby varietals can also be easier on digestion than their tougher, more fibrous siblings.

Microgreens, often used as a garnish at high-end restaurants, are the most expensive of the pack, due to their extremely short shelf life. Often just a week or two off the farm, these itty-bitty greens have been shown to have anywhere from three to six times the amount of nutrients in comparison to their more mature relations. To gain the nutrients but avoid the price tag that accompanies them, microgreens can be grown quite simply in your windowsill for a fraction of the cost and are abundant in antioxidants, phytonutrients, minerals, vitamins, and enzymes.

PAPAYAS

Papayas are a unique fruit in that they also contain a protein-digesting enzyme papain. Papain is often isolated and found in the supplement department of health stores as a digestive aid, or support for indigestion. Papayas are high in magnesium, which is a natural relaxant for the heart and smooth muscles, including the intestines. This quality helps waste move through the system. Although they should be supportive of beautiful skin in their own right, they have also made their way to the top of the list for most likely to be genetically modified, meaning they are often GMOs.

This is quite disappointing, considering GMO foods are modified for desirable traits, including pesticide and herbicide resistance, improved shelf life, and to be able to stand up to harsh climates. While this sounds fine and dandy, the process of genetic medication can include mutating, deleting, or inserting new genes, often from different organisms! This means that a tomato can actually have the genes from a pig!

Not all papayas are GMO. Organic produce is not allowed to be labeled "organic" if it is GMO. At the moment, Hawaiian papayas are considered GMO, while papayas from Mexico and the Caribbean are not.

PARSLEY

Often used as plate décor at swanky restaurants or sprinkled as a garnish in various dishes, parsley is easily overlooked and taken for granted. However, it's a good source of the electrolyte potassium, which is useful in maintaining and regulating the amount of water the body holds. It is also a good source of calcium and magnesium, alkaline minerals that promote healthy bones and an ideal blood pH for beautiful skin.

A superior food for detoxification, parsley supports the healthy functioning of the bladder, kidneys, and liver. It is also said to have both diuretic and blood-purifying properties, having been used by natural and holistic health practitioners to flush heavy metals from the blood. Parsley may also be helpful in eliminating harmful byproducts of meat consumption, like uric acid, which can create inflammation and pain.

A good source of antioxidants, both the leaves and the stems can be juiced into vegetable juices or smoothies. Because the stems are tough, fibrous, and difficult to digest, it is best to only use the leaves chopped and tossed into salads.

PINEAPPLE

Pineapples are a fascinating tropical fruit that are often recognized for their high vitamin C content. Vitamin C is an essential water-soluble antioxidant that must be obtained through the diet. It is the main ingredient in the production of collagen and is necessary for strong bones, teeth, muscles, and a youthful, glowing complexion.

Best eaten when just freshly sliced, and on an empty stomach (as with all fruits), pineapple contains the enzyme bromelain, a powerful digestive aid with anti-inflammatory and cleansing properties.

Often isolated for supplementation, bromelain is one of the protein-digesting enzymes highly regarded for its ability to improve and enhance digestion. If you find that eating too much pineapple leaves your tongue feeling sore, there is good reason: bromelain is so effective in breaking down proteins it can be used as a natural meat tenderizer.

As an anti-inflammatory, it is prescribed to treat joint inflammation in rheumatoid arthritis, as well as to combat swelling after post-traumatic stress. These anti-inflammatory, antiswelling, and digestion-enhancing qualities make it an excellent fruit to enjoy.

In addition, pineapples also contain sulfur, which has been shown to promote the elimination of toxins from the blood and lymphatic system. Daily detoxification and cleansing are necessary obligations for beautiful and radiant skin. When wastes sit within the body, the resulting disaster allows toxic residue and matter to be swept up back into the bloodstream and force the liver and vital organs to deal with excess stress instead of cell regeneration.

Note: Pineapple is also rich in sugar. If you are suffering from acne, or believe that you have candida, it is wise to reduce and eliminate all fruit from the diet until you have improved your digestion and lifestyle choices.

RADISHES

Radishes are a uniquely spicy root vegetable, rich in alkaline minerals that support natural detoxification. Radishes have a diuretic effect on the body and are therefore helpful in the normal functioning of the kidneys and bladder.

Radishes can be juiced or shredded into raw salads. Dr. Norman W. Walker considered radishes to be helpful in flushing excess mucus from the body, which can prevent waste from leaving the system.

ROMAINE

Oh how I love romaine. It is one of the easiest greens to introduce into the Standard American Diet because it is so mild in flavor and slightly sweet. Most commonly used in the Caesar salad, romaine can be dismissed by kale aficionados for not being green enough. I had an older gentleman client once call me up to ask if he could substitute iceberg lettuce for romaine because it was much cheaper. "Heavens, no!" I told him. "We want you to be nourishing the body with nutrients or you won't feel satisfied." Unlike iceberg lettuce, which is practically void of nutrients, romaine is a good source of age-defying vitamin A (beta-carotene) and C, as well as vitamin K and folate. It serves as a viable source of some of the B vitamins and is considered anti-inflammatory, with a greater percentage of its fatty acids coming from omega-3s.

Romaine is also a wonderful source of alkaline minerals and electrolytes. My love for romaine has as much to do with its seductive crunch as it does its versatility. I use the leaves as sandwich wraps and in smoothies. In fact, I save the bottom portion of the head for my juice. I will even happily enjoy romaine leaves with a sprinkle of sea salt if I am on the move, or a drizzle of raw honey if I am looking for something sweet. Each bite packs in fiber and makes it easy to get in that raw salad prior to enjoying cooked foods.

SEA VEGETABLES AND SEAWEED

Believe it or not, vegetables of the sea are some of the most potent sources of nutrients available. A good source of protein, iodine, and bone-strengthening calcium, blood-oxygenating iron, and electrolyte-enhancing potassium, sea vegetables pack a powerful punch. Among the most readily available in grocery and health stores are dulse, kombu, and my personal favorite, nori.

Nori is one of the most commonly used and recognized sea vegetables, especially for those familiar with sushi. Each dark green nori sheet is roughly 1 gram of protein and an excellent source of age-reversing vitamin A, calcium, iron, and iodine. I use nori sheets as I would flour tortillas, wrapping my greens inside, or I have it as a snack when I am looking for a "guilt-free" crunch.

Although both nori and dulse are considered part of the red algae family, dulse is certainly redder in color. Slightly more flavored like the ocean, dulse is an excellent source of iron, calcium, and iodine. Usually available in a flaked form, it can be sprinkled over salads or used in soups and with steamed greens as a mineral-rich salt replacement.

The body needs iodine, an essential trace mineral, for natural hormone function. Iodine deficiency can cause serious medical problems and a number of issues not limited to weight gain, low energy, and depression. To solve iodine deficiency due to a lack of this mineral in our inorganic soils, iodine was added to our salt. However, salt is not something that is lacking in our food industry, and because our culture oversalts our food, the use of table salt, often iodized, can cause us to get far too much iodine in the body, which can lead to skin issues such as acne.

Additionally, table salts are harsh on the body. Processed, bleached white, polished, and often containing other unwanted additives and heavy metals, table salts are not the best way to obtain iodine. Natural sources of iodine make the mineral much more readily available to the body. It can be found in seafood and sea vegetables, as well as onions, mushrooms, and lettuce, depending on the soil content.

Of the seaweeds, kombu is one of the highest in sodium. It is also a great source of calcium and iron, as well as vitamin A and some B vitamins, and can be a mineral-rich addition to your favorite soups. It is part of the brown algae family and considerably rich in both protein and flavor.

SPINACH

Spinach is a great source of iron, which is crucial in healthy circulation, carrying oxygen throughout the body, and giving skin its youthful glow. Coupled with its high proportion of vitamin A in the form of beta-carotene, spinach is a free radical–fighting food, instrumental for clear skin and age reversal.

Also rich in calcium, potassium, and magnesium, spinach contains alkaline minerals that are important for healthy blood and a strong skeletal structure.

Raw spinach is sometimes given a bad reputation due to its high oxalic acid content, which is believed to inhibit calcium absorption. This is still a controversial topic, with very little data to make spinach seem offensive. Oxalic acid aside, spinach is an alkaline food, which is naturally supportive of healthy bones and a superior source of plant-based iron and vitamin K. In combination with a diet of a variety of greens, supported by a lifestyle that enhances the digestion and assimilation of foods and nutrients, raw spinach is still beneficial. There has been no evidence to support the detriment of it to our health.

That being said, if raw spinach is of concern, collards, kale, and other dark leafy greens are other excellent sources of vitamin A and calcium and can be used to support a beautiful complexion.

SPROUTS

Much like microgreens, sprouts are among the most nutrient-rich foods we can add into our diet. Sprouts are little seedlings that have just started to grow. Each seedling is equipped with an abundance of potent nutrients and amino acids that are designed to help feed and nourish the seedling into a strong, mature plant. Thinking that it is safe to grow, a seedling will begin to rapidly multiply the nutrients needed for growth. When we eat these germinating seedlings, we are eating the plant at the time of its life when nutrients are the most abundant.

A sprout is virtually a little burst of life and energy and is instrumental in cell regeneration and a beautiful and healthy complexion. Sprouts come in many varieties, including broccoli sprouts, alfalfa, sunflower sprouts, and onion sprouts, to name a few. They can be easily and cost-effectively grown in your windowsill at home. My personal favorites are onion sprouts, as they add a tinge of spiciness to my salads, as well as sunflower sprouts, which I use when hosting springtime lunches and dinners for my clients.

Enjoy sprouts on top of your salads and in smoothies, and be sure to rinse them prior to use.

SWEET POTATOES

Sweet potatoes get their gorgeous color from beta-carotene, which is converted into vitamin A in the body. Often confused with or used interchangeably to describe yams, sweet potatoes are the less starchy "twin" available to us in the United States. Although very similar, sweet potatoes are richer in beta-carotene than their looka-likes, making them a valuable addition to youthful skin, promoting cell regeneration and preventing free radical formation.

Sweet potatoes are also a good source of iron, potassium, vita-min C, and a fairly good source of some of the B vitamins. Cate-gorically, they are considered a high-quality starch, easily digested by most, and a great alternative to grains. Unlike white potatoes, sweet potatoes can be juiced, scrubbed and eaten raw like a carrot, or baked.

When digested, sweet potatoes can supply the body and skin with immune-boosting vitamins and antioxidants, unlike their col-orless counterparts. Their fiber-to-sugar ratio is ideal; instead of spiking our blood sugar levels, as is the case with many starches, pastas and white potatoes included, they keep us balanced. Similar to carrots, sweet potatoes support a youthful, clear complexion.

TOMATOES

Tomatoes are a fruit but can be treated as a neutral vegetable for our purposes in Food Combining (see page 194). A more acid fruit, tomatoes are a hydrating source of electrolytes and the alkalizing minerals calcium and magnesium.

Eaten fresh and raw as a snack, they can be alkalizing. Cooked or combined with grains, they can become acid-forming, inflamma-tory, and irritating to the joints, intestines, and kidneys.

When working with a client who is looking to clear their acne or other topical skin disorder, I recommend tomatoes since they can be tolerated in the diet, often more easily than fruit. This means they are also an OK food to leave in the diet when focusing on rid-ding the body of yeasts like candida.

Tomatoes are red due to the antioxidant pigment lycopene, which also gives watermelon its delightful color. Lycopene acts as an antioxidant in the body, and is therefore beneficial in protecting against aging caused by free radical damage. I include tomatoes in this section because baby or cherry tomatoes can be an excellent remedy for fruit cravings!

YOUNG THAI COCONUT

Not all coconuts are created equal. Young Thai coconuts are white cone-shaped coconuts, cut from their larger green shell, sold in specialty grocers. These coconuts contain both a tender, mild-tasting white meat and a sweet, electrolyte-rich clear water. It is these coconuts that should be associated with the coconut water craze.

Mature coconuts, the ones we often associate with hanging from a tree, are furry, brown, and round. They contain a much heartier, denser meat, much more similar to that of a nut. The liquid inside is a murky white, and is generally referred to as the "milk." The body treats these coconuts like nuts, and they are more challenging to digest than the softer meat of a young coconut.

When meeting with a new client, I will often mention the potential benefit of coconut in the diet, as an example for a healthy fat. The initial response I get is usually not one concerning fat content, but rather some look of disgust or pleasure. Often, clients think I am talking about the scraggly, dehydrated, often artificial pieces that are used in the food industry. Regardless, I have found clients have either a strong positive or negative relationship with these coconuts.

Young Thai coconuts, on the other hand, contain a flimsy meat, much more delicate in flavor. It can be used as a dairy alternative to make cream, ice cream, icing, pudding, desserts, and sauces in place of dairy products. The meat itself is a quality source of protein and fiber, and also is thought to have antibacterial and antifungal properties due to its lauric acid content. Coconut meat is a saturated fat, meaning that it is more stable to the molecular change a fat undergoes when heated, and less susceptible to free radical formation, which accelerates disease, cell damage, and aging. Although any heat applied to fat is not ideal, I recommend using coconut oil when sautéing something plant-based or organic butter when cooking something animal-based. Personally, I would much rather steam my food and add a dash of olive oil or raw avocado flesh after cooking.

The saturated fat in coconut is fine when eaten in moderation; indeed, all fats should be eaten in moderation to avoid creating excess stress on the liver. The term "saturated" is only a cause for concern when the original source of saturated fat is from a processed or animal food, one that by law creates inflammation and which the body struggles to break down. Coconut is considered anti-inflammatory and keeps the skin supple and hydrated. It is naturally cholesterol-free.

Coconut water is nature's sports drink. While I do not consider coconut water to be beneficial for those who may have candida-related problems due to its higher concentration of sugar, its high level of electrolytes makes it one of the most hydrating beverages we can choose.

ZUCCHINI

Inexpensive, versatile, and an excellent source of fiber, zucchini and yellow squash make it simple to pack many of the B vitamins into your diet. They also are a great source of immune and collagen-boosting vitamin C.

Zucchini makes for an excellent substitute for pasta dishes. Mild enough to be masked by marinara and other Italian sauces, and just "starchy" enough to pass for white pasta or rice noodles, zucchini offers a variety of alkaline minerals while helping you transition from hard-to-digest noodle dishes to energy-enhancing pseudo-Italian and Asian cuisine. A natural source of sugar and a splendid source of fiber, zucchini helps you feel fuller faster without the spike in blood sugar levels and inflammation that white starches cause the body.

Invest in a spiralizer or perforated vegetable peeler to create fiber-rich zucchini noodles that are also mineral-rich, alkaline, and anti-inflammatory, and that will not leave you crashing or craving sugars.

As of 2013, zucchini was added to the Dirty Dozen Plus list (page 80) and also has a high likelihood of being genetically modified. For that reason, choose organic zucchini or zucchini from a vendor at your local farmer's market that you know uses organic farming practices.

Build a Better Salad

Choose your green base from Column 1. Greens are an essential part of any life-sustaining meal and can and should be enjoyed in abundance at every meal, in any and every variety. You can keep it simple with spinach, but get creative with mixed greens such as arugula, baby kale, and chopped romaine.

Choose your raw salad additions from Column 2. Fill up on these first and use the remaining additional options to add more density to your salad if needed.

Choose your protein of choice from Column 3. Regardless of common belief, each of these items contains protein, but not all of them digest well when combined together at the same meal.

Column 4 includes options that digest well with the "protein" you have chosen. For instance, columns one and two are ideal for any salad, but once you choose a protein, you should only choose additional items that correspond with that protein. Certain ingredients will overlap, but other ingredients should never be combined together.

Column 5 addresses healthy dressing options and alternatives to bottled dressings. They are simple and serve to enhance the flavor of your salad, instead of mask it. It is important to avoid bottled dressings, as they often contain added sugars, cheap oils, additives, and additional ingredients that do not serve us well and can make a relatively nutrient-dense salad unhealthy.

In other words, a salad or meal with quinoa may be added to a salad with avocado, but never to a salad with grilled chicken, fish, cheese, or nuts/seeds/dried fruit.

Build a Better Salad

1. Greens	2. Veggies	3. Proteins	4. Protein Additions	5. Dressings
· Arugula · Baby kale · Baby romaine · Bok choy · Collards · Kale · Mâche · Mixed greens · Romaine · Spinach **Herbs:** · Fresh cilantro · Fresh parsley · Fresh basil	**Raw Veggies:** · Scallions · Red, orange, yellow bell peppers · Shredded beets · Shredded carrots · Corn · Cherry tomatoes · Tomatoes · Jalapeños · Sun-dried tomatoes · Zucchini · Broccoli sprouts · Sunflower sprouts · Olives · Garlic **Lightly Steamed:** · Broccoli · Cauliflower · Zucchini **Cooked:** · Artichokes · Roasted cauliflower · Roasted beets · Grilled, roasted, or baked zucchini · Mushrooms · Roasted garlic	**Avocado:** · ½ cup guacamole, 1 whole small avocado, or ½ medium/large avocado **Quinoa:** · ½–1 cup **Cheese:** · ¼ cup shredded (Use Parmesan, goat feta, or sheep Manchego) **Fish** · 3–4 oz. **Raw Nuts/ Seeds & Dried Fruit** · ¼ cup seeds/ nuts, ⅛ cup dried fruit **Organic Chicken or Grass-fed Beef** · 3–4 oz.	· Baked sweet potato · Scoop of quinoa · Scoop of brown rice · Handful baked corn tortilla chips · Cooked corn or peas · ¼ cup guaca-mole, or 1 small avocado · Baked sweet potato · Baked winter squash · Cooked corn or peas · Grilled chicken · Shrimp · Roasted or steamed vegetables · Roasted, grilled, or steamed vegetables · *Avoid*: all fresh fruit, animal products, grains, and beans · Shredded Parmesan, sheep, Manchego, or goat feta	**Base:** · Avocado · Olive oil · Flax oil **Acid:** · Lemon juice · Lime juice · Raw apple cider vinegar · Raw coconut aminos · Low-sodium, gluten-free tamari **Seasonings:** · Sea salt · Honey **Spices that add warmth:** · Cayenne · Paprika · Cumin · Coriander · Red chili flakes · Dried oregano · Dried basil · Dried thyme · Salt-free Mexican seasoning · Italian blend

Why Go Organic Whenever Possible?

Remember, our skin is the backup organ for the liver and kidney. Toxic residues specifically burden our liver, and what it cannot neutralize or eliminate effectively may come through the pores or be stored and damage cells. Pesticides used in conventional farming practices invite free radical formation, create excess inflammation, poison the blood, and create unnecessary stress on our vital organs. The more we invite these substances into the body, the more we invite acidity into the organs, tissue, fat cells, and blood. This type of environment becomes ideal for bacteria and disease, and makes us highly susceptible to external allergies and rapid aging. Additionally, many pesticides used in conventional farming have been shown to be carcinogenic.

Understandably, buying organically grown produce may not always fit into every budget, but there are several items you should try to avoid when possible if they aren't certified organic or grown by farmers in your area using organic practices. These foods are taken from the 2013 list created by the Environmental Working Group (www.ewg.org).

Dirty Dozen Plus

1. Apples
2. Celery
3. Cherry tomatoes
4. Cucumbers
5. Grapes
6. Peppers
7. Nectarines
8. Peaches
9. Potatoes

10. Spinach
11. Strawberries
12. Greens: kale, collards, romaine
13. Zucchini and yellow squash

With this list in mind, I would much rather my clients include inorganic vegetables in their diet than not at all, which leads me to our next topic: "What if I cannot afford to buy all organic?"

Let me be frank. Although there are inorganic foods I would rather not purchase when given the choice, I like to rephrase the question instead and ask my clients, "If you are not buying these organic berries because of price, what are you eating instead?" While I do not advocate the regular consumption of inorganic berries, for instance, I often find that instead of looking for another fruit or wholesome option, like a banana, orange, or seasonal fruit, it gives us an excuse to consume something entirely more processed. For instance, instead of inorganic berries, one is likely to opt for a "whole-grain cereal with a milk or a milk alternative," or commercial "sweet potato chips." These foods offer little to no nutritional value on their own and usually contain a considerable amount of additives and/or are highly processed. I find that often the good can outweigh the bad when we are considering adding more fruits and vegetables into our diet in place of other, less wholesome options.

Purchase organic greens when you can, especially when juicing. Make organic and organically raised greens a priority, but don't let it be a reason or cause for not eating fresh or frozen produce in general.

My suggestion is to look in the frozen sections of grocery stores and wholesalers for organic frozen fruit and greens. Also, stay in the loop with grocery sales and shop seasonally and locally, which reduces the amount of money distributors must pay for the transportation of food. This all sounds like common sense, but if what is keeping you from buying produce is the "organic" stamp of approval, and the price tag that comes with it, then please place that notion aside and purchase other produce outside of the Dirty Dozen list.

Foods that have harder exteriors, like oranges, grapefruits, bananas, and avocados, are considered less likely to absorb more external pesticides. The EWG 2013 "Clean 15" is a list of fruits and vegetables with the least trace pesticides. This means they can more safely be purchased in their conventional, non-organic-certified forms.

The Clean 15

1. Asparagus
2. Avocados
3. Cabbage
4. Cantaloupe
5. Sweet corn
6. Eggplant
7. Grapefruit
8. Kiwi
9. Mangos
10. Mushrooms
11. Onions
12. Papayas
13. Pineapples
14. Sweet peas, frozen
15. Sweet potatoes

The detox plan in this book does not place an emphasis on fruit due to their high levels of sugar, though otherwise they are great in moderation but can feed toxic yeasts like candida when topical skin disorders, such as acne, eczema, and rashes are a cause for concern.

WHAT ABOUT DINING OUT?

I love the dining-out experience, but I realize I cannot always be the one to dictate where my friends and I go. I do go out to dinner and enjoy big green salads, which are not always organic or local. But what would be the alternative? No salad? I assure you, I would not feel so grand if I enjoyed a bowl of rice instead. How do I navigate? I try my best to plan ahead, making sure that before I leave to head out, I have had something alkaline (and organic if possible) so I am not entering a land unknown and starving. I also always check the menu online. If I am a guest for dinner, I always offer to bring a salad and casually insert that I am vegetarian and would love to bring something that everyone can enjoy.

Dining out and social outings should be enjoyable. Enjoy the company you are with and don't sweat the small stuff. If you are enjoying that big leafy green salad with veggies, olive oil, and fresh squeezed lemon, that is great, despite the fact that it may not be a full-on organic meal. An organic meal with toxic company is not "organic" either.

Use the "Best Options When Dining Out" chart on page 198 to help guide you through placing an order at your favorite restaurant. The following chapter, "Food Combining and Foods to Enjoy," will help you better understand in detail why some of these choices are so.

CHAPTER 4

Food Combining & Foods to Enjoy

Digestion is an ongoing theme throughout this book, and it's one of the most important factors in achieving a youthful, glowing complexion.

In order to almost effortlessly improve digestion, food must provide quick, sustainable nourishment and be "relatively" quick to exit. This is not difficult when your diet is rich in wholesome, plant-based foods, for reasons that have already been discussed.

In fact, aside from ridding your diet of unnatural and processed foods, effortlessly improving digestion can be as easy as enjoying "like foods" with "like foods," or food combining.

Food combining is one of the simplest, healthiest, and most natural ways to improve nutritional absorption, maximize digestion, and cleanse the digestive tract of the unwanted substances and matter causing the skin to age, blemish, and suffer.

In the simplest of explanations, food can be separated into five groups based on how they are digested:

- Fresh fruits and fruit and vegetable juices
- Vegetables

- "Wholesome" starches (not to be confused with refined grains), including beans, legumes, and lentils
- Animal proteins
- Nuts, seeds, and dried fruit

These groups represent the most common types of food we may encounter on an everyday basis. They do not include junk foods, highly processed foods, or fast foods, as those are unfit for *any* body. (Packaged pastries, for instance, are not considered a wholesome "starch," and deli meat is not considered a "healthful" source of animal protein).

This does not mean that you can only eat vegetables for lunch and nuts for dinner. These groups are designed to give you a foundation for recognizing different food groups on an everyday basis. Some groups combine together perfectly—for instance, steamed broccoli with organic butter and a grilled chicken breast or baked fish—while others you should avoid eating together at meals—for instance, nuts and animal protein.

The purpose of eating within these categories is to increase the rate at which nutrients are extracted, assimilated, digested, and then excreted. In other words, the quicker foods are to nourish and exit the digestive tract, the less likely they are to become a detriment to skin. The enzymes found in living plant foods play a major role in the combination and digestion of foods. Foods are categorized based on the stomach environment the enzymes need to work at their most efficient. As you will find, some foods require a more acid environment for digestion, whereas others require a more alkaline environment.

This may sound complicated, but once you understand the different groups, it will become second nature. (For a reference chart, see "The pH of Common Foods" on page 196).

Fresh Fruits and Raw Fruit and Vegetable Juices

With their high water content, fiber, and sugar, fruits should be among the quickest foods to digest. However, fruits should only be consumed on an empty stomach (i.e., at breakfast) and are not to be combined with other foods, especially cooked or denser foods. When combined with other foods (which take longer to digest than fruits), eaten as a dessert (after a meal), or enjoyed as an afternoon snack, the high water and sugar content will cause the fresh fruit to ferment in your stomach. Fermentation causes gas, bloat, and constipation, which slows digestion and encourages the overgrowth of candida. Because fruit and vegetable juices have such a quick transit time as well, all juices should be consumed separately from solid foods, and are thus best consumed for breakfast or prior to breakfast. It is not recommended to drink fresh juice with a meal or even several hours after a meal containing animal products or cooked foods.

I love to explain fruit and food combining to my clientele as the old lady in the express lane of a grocer. Imagine that you are running to a meeting and grabbed lunch at your local market's salad bar. You head to the express line, money ready, on a mission to make your purchase and be on your way. Unfortunately, the little old lady ahead of you has the maximum number of items, forgot an item, and is paying with a check. Regardless of how quickly you could have been on your merry way is insignificant. The old lady is keeping you from realizing your potential.

The takeaway: Eat fruit alone or leave it at home. Due to their quick digestion but also high susceptibility to fermentation in the stomach, fruit is best consumed for breakfast, as are fruit and vegetables juices. The groups below are separated based on how well various fruits digest together.

Melons

Melons are a unique fruit in that they are almost entirely made up of water and therefore digest the quickest when eaten alone or prior to denser fruits (fruits from other categories).

- Watermelon
- Cantaloupe
- Honeydew

Low-Sugar Fruits

- Blueberries
- Strawberries
- Raspberries
- Blackberries
- Apples (use green apples when juicing, as they are lower in sugar)

Sub-Acidic Fruits (fruits that digest fine together when grouped)

- Apples
- Pears
- Peaches
- Plums
- Papayas
- Mangos

Acidic Fruits (unrelated to pH)

- Oranges
- Pineapples
- Grapefruits
- Tangerines
- Clementines

Simple Fruits
- Bananas (ripe)
- Grapes
- Persimmons

Exceptions
- With the exception of bananas and avocados, fruit should be eaten alone or left alone.

EXCEPTIONS TO THE FRUIT RULE

Bananas: They contain less water than most fruits and can be eaten with vegetables, avocados, starches, nuts, and dried fruit. They should never be eaten with animal products.

However, bananas, as with all fruits, are also very high in sugar. If you suffer from acne, or any sort of dermatitis, fruits should be temporarily eliminated from your diet. If this seems too "extreme," very low-sugar fruits can be added as breakfast-only items. These include green apples and berries. Unfortunately, even natural sugars cause destruction when candida is present.

Dried Fruit: Dried fruit, although more concentrated in sugar than fresh fruit, no longer contains the water that would have helped guide it through the digestive system quickly. Not ideal for candida, dried fruits will be discussed in greater detail later in this chapter.

Cooked Fruit: Cooking fruit concentrates natural sugars and destroys beneficial enzymes and beneficial properties, including water-soluble vitamins and antioxidants. I do not recommend eating cooked fruits unless they are enjoyed on their own as a warming breakfast during cooler months (for example, baked organic apple slices with cinnamon as a breakfast after having juice and/or a green smoothie).

Green Smoothies: Blending pulverizes and breaks down the tough plant cellulose, or fibers, of fruits and vegetables. The act of blending is in effect helping to predigest the food. Blended plant foods can be much easier for individuals to digest because the majority of the work has been done for the stomach and shortens the amount of time the food has to remain waiting for transit to the small intestine. A green smoothie is an alkaline combination of fiber-containing, low-sugar fruits like bananas, dark leafy greens, herbs, green vegetables, and water. Fresh juice and green smoothies are both beneficial, but serve different purposes in the diet.

Vegetables

High in natural plant fibers (cellulose), uncooked or very lightly cooked vegetables not only provide incredible nourishment but also sweep the colon of unwanted waste and matter. When "living" foods are heated at high temperatures, beneficial nutrients and enzymes are destroyed. When these vegetables are living and vibrant with nutrients and enzymes, these delicious "colon sweepers" are considered neutral and can be eaten and combined with any of the listed categories except the first: fruits.

Some vegetables change chemically once cooked. For instance, carrots and corn become more starchy and concentrated in sugar when they are heated. Carrots and corn are not considered neutral once cooked. The chart on page 194 will help you to better determine which vegetables these are. Note that raw vegetables, though often touted for their "raw healing properties," are not always superior to lightly cooked vegetables. Cruciferous vegetables like broccoli, cauliflower, and Brussels sprouts are harder to digest raw because they have a lower water content than other vegetables like zucchini and squash. Lightly steaming these vegetables will loosen the plant fibers and make them easier to digest.

Neutral (low-starch) vegetables, especially raw leafy greens, should be eaten with every meal and even more specifically at meals that are devoid of enzymes and/or may be difficult to digest on their own. Raw and lightly steamed vegetables and their juices can be wonderful sources of food enzymes, which also help to digest foods that do not contain their own enzymes, such as animal proteins (meat, poultry, most cheese, fish, eggs, yogurt) and heavier starches (breads, pastas, flours, potatoes, etc.).

Leafy Greens (Highest pH)
- Arugula
- Kale
- Mâche
- Microgreens
- Romaine
- Spinach
- Sprouts
- Sunflower sprouts

Lightly Steamed
- Asparagus
- Bok choy
- Broccoli
- Brussels sprouts
- Cauliflower
- Zucchini
- Summer squash

Lower pH
- Baked eggplant
- Roasted cauliflower
- Lightly grilled vegetables

Starches

Starches are long "complex" chains of simple sugars, or glucose. They are also referred to as complex carbohydrates, or "carbs," though most foods that contain sugar also contain carbohydrates. Starches vary in their ratios of protein, gluten, water, fiber, fat, and sugar. In this sense, starches are not all created equal and they can be arranged in a hierarchy—some are less processed, more nutrient-dense, and ultimately easier to digest than others. Natural, unprocessed starches can be beneficial, while processed, heated, and treated starches create "sludgelike" waste that inevitably sticks to the walls of the digestive tract like a paste and invites disease.

Highly processed and refined starches, like white hamburger buns, cheese doodles, and donuts, have zero place in a healthful diet. Processed foods can claim that they are made with whole grains when they *include* whole-grain ingredients in *addition* to processed ingredients. Most grains, for instance, are generally processed and stripped of their nutrients. These processed grains affect blood sugar levels, thereby affecting energy levels and inviting sugar-related problems like adrenal fatigue and hormonal issues. There are many types of grains, including rice, quinoa, buckwheat, amaranth, millet, Kamut, spelt, barley, rye, wheat, and oats, among others. As with all starches, some of these grains are more easily digested than others often because they are less processed than others.

Minimally processed starches (baked corn tortilla chips, rice cakes, gluten-free pasta, rice crackers) can be great transitional foods to enjoy as you experiment with this new lifestyle.

Avoid white starches like flours, pastas, white rice crackers, cookies, all popcorn, etc. This also includes products that misleadingly claim to be "whole grain." Most foods claiming "whole-grain" contain gluten. Gluten digests like it sounds, sticking to the body like "glue" and causing irritation and inflammation. These foods are converted into sugar, feed candida, and add to the "sticky" sludgelike paste in the body. Brown rice can be an acceptable gluten-free food to transition with, but rice tends to be "gluey" also and is not quick to exit the body, nor does it provide an abundance of nutrients.

Popcorn is particularly difficult to digest, as popcorn kernels get stuck in the diverticula (nooks and crannies) of the intestinal tissue. Popcorn is a perfect example of how the expression "calories in" does not equal "calories out." Although air-popped popcorn is very low in calories and high in fiber, it is also impossible for the body to completely break down and digest. Additionally, popcorn is very low in nutrients. Instead of being a snack that also serves the body, popcorn is a filler food that slows digestion and offers little if any benefit. Although seemingly harmless and diet-friendly, buttered and salted popcorn is not a healthy choice for beautiful skin or digestion.

Sprouted grain products are generally the least processed of all the traditional bread items, including wheat and white breads. Sprouted grains grow within young plants and are considered "living" complete proteins. Minimally processed and rarely "fortified," their nutrients are much more prolific and therefore better digested and assimilated. Sprouted grain products (like the "Food For Life" product line) are in a growing number of grocers and can be readily found in the freezer section of specialty food stores. Adding fresh slices of avocado to a minimally processed (and preferably sprouted) piece of toasted grain bread can help it "move" through the digestive tract for a quicker exit.

In addition to grains, cooked carrots and corn, root vegetables like sweet potatoes, white potatoes, and winter squashes (acorn, butternut, pumpkin, kabocha) all fall under the starch category.

Starches combine well with neutral vegetables, but none of the other food categories, with the exception of bananas, avocados, and young Thai coconuts, which contain less water and are less likely to ferment. Although technically a fruit, avocados have a very unique profile—high in fat, protein, and fiber. Avocados are actually quite beneficial to the digestive system, providing it with the "lubricating" qualities of a laxative and an abundance of nutrients. Avocados digest best with foods in the starch category. Avocados should never be combined with animal products (dairy and meat), nuts, or seeds; they can be combined with bananas and dried fruit. Similarly, the white "meat" of a young Thai coconut is a healthy source of fat that can be beneficial in moderation. It can be combined with fruit or nuts.

LOVE GRAINS?

Gluten-free alternatives to white and wheat breads such as quinoa, millet, amaranth, and buckwheat are among the most readily digestible and most alkaline grains. Kamut and spelt grains are also considerably less processed than and preferred to "whole grain" foods. Rye and barley are two of the most acid-forming whole grains in the bunch and should be avoided altogether, in addition to wheat and white bread. Rice and popcorn, though traditionally thought of as "healthful" and naturally gluten-free, are not ideal for beautiful skin because they are low in nutrients and slow to digest.

Cooked quinoa and millet are delicious alternatives to bread, rice, couscous, and barley, and can be a satisfyingly nourishing way to get the carbohydrates your body is used to receiving without breaking the bank or causing inflammation. Heat them on the stovetop according to package instruction with onions, peppers, and your favorite seasonings, or sweeten quinoa and millet with stevia, cinnamon, and a touch of coconut milk as a breakfast option.

In general, here are a few good rules of thumb to keep in mind when cooking grains:

- Starches should never be combined with animal products, with the exception of a minimal amount of organic butter for flavor.
- Starches should not be combined with nuts, seeds, or dried fruit. All grains should *always* be consumed with greens and steamed vegetables to aid digestion.
- Grains, unless living and sprouted, lack the enzymes needed to help digest them completely and properly.

THE BEST "STARCHES": A HIERARCHY

Here is a break down, beginning with the most nourishing and beautifying "starches."

- Avocado (technically a fatty fruit)
- Young Thai coconuts (technically a fatty fruit)
- Root vegetables, like baked sweet potatoes and seasonal squashes (spaghetti, acorn, kabocha, etc.)
- Millet, quinoa, amaranth, buckwheat
- Baked potatoes, although not an ideal source of nourishment, can be a good option for those highly sensitized to all gluten, and especially great for those on a budget or who dine out frequently. They also may be easier for some to digest than rice and sprouted grains because they are less processed.
- Brown rice can be a good gluten-free alternative for many, especially when trying to avoid all forms of gluten.
- Sprouted grains (look for spelt and kamut products) are considered the most processed in this group, but may be easier for some to digest than brown rice. Ideally, the less processed an item is, the easier it is for the body to break down and use.

BEANS, LEGUMES, AND LENTILS

Beans, legumes, and lentils are all in the same family and commonly referred to under the umbrella term "beans." This includes all forms, colors, and varieties: kidney, black, pinto, white, cannellini, red, brown, green and yellow lentils, as well as chickpeas (garbanzo beans), lima beans, split peas, and edamame (soybeans), to name a few.

This category is unique in that these foods naturally contain high levels of both starch and protein, making them nature's "whoops"—a food that, on its own, is a challenge for our digestive system to break down. It is for this reason that people tend to experience flatulence and acid reflux from beans. It is also why there is a well-marketed over-the-counter medication called Beano to help ease digestive discomfort.

As mentioned in the section on soy (a bean), beans contain phytic acid and can actually pull nutrients from our bodies, often those such as magnesium, calcium, zinc, and iron, minerals needed for radiant skin. In addition to phytic acid, most beans contain enzyme inhibitors. These prevent our bodies from being able to break down the bean and can be quite irritating to the intestines.

Why all of the problems? Beans are designed to withstand unpredictable environments and to keep the little bean from sprouting until conditions are good enough for them to grow. As with grains, the phytic acid in the bean is designed to leach onto minerals that will help nourish it and support its growth. This may be ideal for the bean, but not for our body.

Though not ideal for beautiful skin, legumes are an inexpensive form of plant protein and also a fantastic transitional food for those used to heartier meals involving meat, because they are more alkaline than animal meat. The smaller the bean, the easier it is for our body to digest. Lentils are thus our best choice for consumption.

Sprouting beans and lentils can help to ease digestion by deactivating the enzyme inhibitors.

Although a category in their own right, beans, lentils, and legumes will combine better with the starch category and can therefore work transitionally in an animal-free lentil "burrito" along with an abundance of leafy greens and steamed vegetables. Legumes should never be combined with other concentrated proteins, such as nuts, seeds, or any animal products.

Starchy Vegetables
- Cooked carrots
- Cooked peas
- Cooked corn
- Sweet potatoes
- White potatoes

Winter Squash
- Acorn squash
- Butternut
- Kabocha
- Spaghetti squash

Gluten-Free Grains (most alkaline)
- Amaranth
- Buckwheat
- Millet
- Quinoa

Gluten-Free (but digests with difficulty)
- Brown rice

Grains containing gluten
- Kamut
- Spelt
- Wheat

Other
- Avocado
- Young Thai coconut

Exceptions
- Avocados can be combined with dried fruit (but never nuts).
- Young Thai coconuts can be combined with nuts, seeds, and dried fruit.

Indulgences
- Coconut-based ice creams (dairy-free)
- Frozen or ripe bananas

Legumes
- Lentils and other beans (including edamame) are best consumed with neutral vegetables. If you are new to food combining, you can get away with treating them as a starch. I recommend limiting the consumption of this category to decrease gas and digestive discomfort.

Animal Proteins

As previously discussed, human beings were not designed to eat the amount of animal products that are made so readily available to us today.

Meat takes a much longer time to pass through our system than fruits and vegetables, and it becomes very susceptible to putrefaction. When something putrefies, it decays. When a person who enjoys a regular intake of meat is ill (or if they have endured traumatic stress), their breath will smell putrid! This is because their body is trying to detoxify itself in order to heal and the foul smell is part of the process. You will never see a sick animal eating meat. If they eat at all, they will graze on vegetables and greens.

Based on a popular diet from the 1960s, the Atkins Diet focused on a diet high in protein and contained virtually no carbohydrates. It revolutionized the diet world; people feasting on burgers and bacon were miraculously becoming slimmer.

But are carbohydrates the bad guys and Atkins the answer? Not so much. In a published study funded by the Atkins Center for Complementary Medicine, 51 obese people on the Atkins Diet were studied over a course of 24 weeks. *The China Study* reported these findings of their study group: "At some point during the twenty-four weeks, twenty-eight subjects (68%) reported constipation, twenty-six (63%) reported bad breath, twenty-one (51%) reported headache, four (10%) noted hair loss, and one woman (1%) reported increased menstrual bleeding." This was after just 24 weeks. Can you imagine their internal organs after a year?

So why did people lose weight on the diet? For starters, "carbohydrates" are virtually eliminated from the diet. This would mean an elimination of donuts, muffins, pastries, breads, pastas, rice, French fries, cereals, etc. These foods are all considerably high in sugar, fat, and gluten and devoid of satisfying nutrients and whole plant fiber. The Atkins Diet most likely works because these Atkins patients are eating in better combinations by eliminating starches, which do not combine well with animal protein; the Atkins Diet mainly consists of animal fats and proteins (protein and protein combine, whereas protein and starch do not). Food combining will favor the occasional steak and steamed broccoli meal over a regular diet of fish and rice.

Animal protein should only be consumed with steamed and raw vegetables (as well as leafy greens). It should never be combined with nuts and seeds, avocado, coconut, soy, or fruit (dried or fresh).

Animal protein may be combined with dairy products like raw goat and sheep cheeses.

Again, if you're interested in learning more about the meat America is consuming, I recommend watching the following documentaries: *Food, Inc.*, *Super Size Me*, and *Forks Over Knives*.

As far as food combining goes, and to simplify things, **dairy** will be considered an animal protein. The most common dairy foods consumed are milk, whipping cream, cheese, ice cream, yogurt, and butter. Cow milk should be eliminated from the diet entirely, along with yogurt and standard ice creams. The more dairy products that are eliminated from the diet, the more rapid and beautifying the results. Acceptable dairy foods to enjoy in moderation are raw goat and sheep cheeses (and if not available, pasteurized goat and sheep are fine), goat's milk ice cream, and organic butter to sauté and season vegetables.

Eggs are considered an animal protein, but I would not recommend combining eggs with meat products, as they are both concentrated in slow-digesting proteins and individually require a lengthy time in the digestive system. Egg whites contain the slow-digesting protein albumin. Albumin is an exceptionally gluey substance. It is hard to break down and can be even slower to digest than red meat. When the goal is to improve digestion, the last thing you should consume for breakfast is an omelet, as it may sit in the stomach for eight hours. (An acceptable dinner may be two to three whole eggs, spinach, chopped peppers, onions, and/or your favorite vegetables with raw goat cheese. Add a side of steamed vegetables for good measure and remember to enjoy a *raw* salad prior to eating any cooked food.)

As mentioned earlier, **fish** is one of the easiest animal proteins to digest. Although we are accustomed to eating fish with rice (a starch) or edamame (a bean), as with sushi, fish is best consumed with greens and vegetables. Strive for eating wild fish that have been sustainably raised.

Combines with: neutral foods only.
- Organic, free-range eggs
- Cheese (goat, sheep, unpasteurized preferred)
- Wild fish
- Organic chicken
- Lamb
- Grass-fed, hormone-free meat

Indulgences
- Laloo's goat milk ice cream (goat-milk)

Nuts, Seeds, and Dried Fruits

Nuts and seeds have a high calorie and fat content for their weight and size. Unlike the fatty but lubricating avocado, nuts and seeds are dense and therefore more difficult to digest. For this reason, they should be eaten in moderation. Nuts and seeds should always be eaten raw and stored in the refrigerator to avoid becoming rancid. Seeds are more alkaline-forming than nuts, and can be easier to digest when they are sprouted. (Sprouting is a whole subject in itself and not one we will cover in this book.) To avoid overeating, one should not consume more than ¼ cup of nuts or seeds at a time. In order to allow enough time to digest, allow for three to four hours to pass before consuming a different category of food.

Dried fruits, while lacking in the fat content that nuts and seeds have, are also dense and contain very little water to help facilitate their movement through the digestive tract. Lower in nutrients but higher in sugar than fresh fruits, dried fruits are also slower to digest and are not ideal when candida is an issue.

In sum, nuts, seeds, and dried fruits are what I like to refer to as "in a pinch meals" instead of just an "anytime" snack.

Combines with: neutral vegetables or alone.

Seeds
- Sunflower
- Pumpkin
- Flax (ground, as the body cannot break down the hard exterior of the whole flax seed)

Nuts
- Almonds
- Almond flour
- Cashews
- Hazelnuts
- Pecans
- Walnuts

Dried Fruit (freeze-dried or dehydrated)
- Mango
- Apple chips
- Raisins

Indulgences
- Coconut-based ice creams (dairy-free)
- Frozen or ripe bananas (coconut-based cereals and bananas combine well with nuts, seeds, and dried fruits)

● ● ● ●

WHAT IS AN "IN-A-PINCH" MEAL?

These are snacks for when you are famished and want to steer clear of the vending machines, donut shops, and fast food restaurants; or they are for three to four hours before dinner and you are not going to make it through class or another meeting. (If you ate animal products for lunch, you must wait at least three hours before changing to a different category of food). In-a-pinch meals are most ideal for when you do not have time to stop for lunch, or a nutrient-dense meal.

In addition to nuts, seeds, and dried fruits, good in-a-pinch snacks include: baby carrots, sliced red bell peppers, cucumber slices, crisp romaine leaves, celery sticks, apples, bananas, a "juice-box-sized" coconut water; coconut or almond milk, home-made trail mix (recipe on page 184), and unprocessed granola without nuts and minimal oil. Keep your snacks in a sealed plastic container or plastic bag if needed.

Your healthiest, most beautifying snack will always be raw veggies. I love chopping up raw sweet potatoes and sprinkling them with sea salt for a crunchy, tasty alternative to carrots.

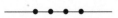

Neutral Foods

Combines with: everything. Enjoy in abundance.

Dressings

- Lemons
- Limes
- Olive oil (cold-pressed)
- Flax oil

- Raw coconut aminos
- Gluten-free tamari

Seasonings

- Spices
- Sea salt
- Himalayan salt
- Stevia

Raw Vegetables

- Carrots
- Celery
- Green beans
- Fennel
- Red, orange, yellow peppers
- Tomatoes
- Sun-dried tomatoes

Exceptions

Due to their high and rough fiber content, it is best to avoid eating the following veggies raw:

- Broccoli
- Brussels sprouts
- Cabbage
- Cauliflower

Indulgences (Enjoy Minimal Consumption)

- Organic 100% butter
- Dark chocolate (70% and above)
- Wine

Quick Food-Combining Recap

Fruit: Disorders of the skin are generally associated with candida (and high sugar intake). It is for this reason that fruit be temporarily eliminated if you're suffering from acne, dark circles, exhaustion, and other disorders commonly associated with adrenal fatigue, including thyroid problems, anxiety, and depression. Fruit should only be consumed on an empty stomach and never combined with other food groups unless being enjoyed in a green smoothie, which is a blended combination of fresh or frozen fruit and greens. Green smoothies should also be consumed on an empty stomach.

Nuts, Seeds, and Dried Fruit: Nuts, seeds, and dried fruits contain very little to virtually no water. They are very dense and should be consumed in moderation (about ¼ cup per serving). Always enjoy nuts and seeds in their raw form, not roasted or with added oils, and avoid dried fruit with additives (no added sugar, sulphurs, etc.). Consume this category by itself, or with greens and the neutral vegetable category.

Exception #1: Bananas can be consumed with raw seeds, nuts, and dried fruit.

Exception #2: Avocados are considered a "starch" but can be consumed with dried fruit and bananas, but never seeds or nuts. They should not be consumed with seeds or nuts because these are two different categories of concentrated fats. When combined, they exhaust the digestive system and steal energy from the body.

Exception #3: Young Thai coconuts can be consumed with nuts, seeds, dried fruit, bananas, and avocados.

Neutral Vegetables: Most raw and lightly steamed vegetables are low in starch and considered neutral, in that they can be combined with all groups. These low-starch vegetables can be consumed with any food category (except fruit). In fact, it is encouraged that they be incorporated at every meal, representing 50 to 95 percent of meal portions. Low-starch vegetables are any vegetable except for those listed below as starches. For our purposes, raw corn and raw carrots can be considered "low-starch" vegetables, whereas cooked corn or carrots are considered starches because cooking them changes their chemical makeup and raises their sugar levels.

Starches: Starches are popularly called "carbohydrates." They can be consumed with other starches, avocados, bananas, young Thai coconuts, and vegetables. Starches are never to be combined with the fruit, nut/seed/dried fruit, or animal flesh categories. Starches include: grains, including rice, potatoes, sweet potatoes, yams, pumpkin, spaghetti or Japanese squash (not to be confused with yellow or zucchini "squashes," which are neutral vegetables), peas, cooked corn and carrots, and legumes.

Animal Protein: This is never to be combined with anything other than "low-starch" vegetables and leafy greens. You would be better off eating more wild or quality fish and vegetables than you would be consuming smaller portions of fish, rice, and vegetables at one meal.

WORST CASE SCENARIOS

These meals are recipes for disaster because not only are they lacking in nutrient-dense greens, but they each include slow-digesting, concentrated foods. When combined together in a meal, the result is an even slower and sluggish metabolism and lower energy.

- Baked potato *(starch)* with cheese *(dairy)*, sour cream *(dairy)*, and bacon bits *(animal protein)*
- Bread *(starch)*, avocado *(starch)*, deli meat *(animal protein)*, mayonnaise
- Whole wheat pasta *(starch)*, with Alfredo sauce *(dairy)*, and shrimp *(animal protein)*

- Cheese *(dairy)* pizza *(starch)* with meat *(animal protein)*
- Fried chicken *(animal protein)* and mashed potatoes *(starch, dairy)*
- Burrito *(starch)* with beans *(legumes)*, rice *(starch)*, chicken *(animal protein)*, guacamole *(starch)*, and cheese *(dairy)*

BETTER CASE SCENARIOS

Breakfast

- Green juice or green smoothie *(neutral greens, vegetables and fruit)*
- Young Thai coconut smoothie (greens, coconut meat, water) *(combines as a starch, with neutral greens)*
- Whole Kamut cereal *(starch)* or gluten-free cereal *(starch)* with coconut milk *(starch)* and freshly sliced banana *(combines as a starch)* sprinkled with cinnamon
- Sprouted or whole-grain or gluten-free toast *(starch)* with fresh avocado *(combines as a starch)* and a sprinkling of sea salt
- Cream of buckwheat *(starch)* with 1 tablespoon grade B maple syrup sprinkled with cinnamon and sea salt
- Chia pudding *(nut, seed, and dried fruit)*
- Cooked quinoa *(combines as a starch)* with coconut milk *(starch)* and 1 tablespoon grade B maple syrup

Lunch

- Chopped salad *(neutral)* with fresh guacamole *(starch)*, pico de gallo *(neutral)*, baked blue corn tortilla chips *(starch)*, steamed or lightly sautéed fajita vegetables *(neutral)*, side of quinoa *(starch)*
- Massaged kale *(neutral)* and avocado salad *(starch)*, sweet potato *(starch)* with coconut butter or organic butter

(maximum 1 tablespoon) *(neutral)*, steamed or lightly sau-téed vegetables *(neutral)*

- Baby greens *(neutral)* with fresh-squeezed lemon juice and avocado *(starch)*, lentil soup *(starch)*, steamed vegetables *(neutral)*
- Baby greens *(neutral)* with grilled or steamed vegetables *(neutral)* and ⅓ cup shaved Manchego cheese or goat's milk feta cheese *(animal protein)*
- Baby greens *(neutral)* with fresh-squeezed lemon juice and goat's milk feta cheese *(animal protein)*, grilled chicken or salmon *(animal protein)*, steamed vegetables *(neutral)*

Dinner

See above, and also consider the following:

- Zucchini noodles *(neutral)* with avocado cream sauce *(starch)* or marinara *(neutral)* and shaved Manchego cheese *(animal protein)*, fresh basil, steamed vegetables *(neutral)*
- Grilled salmon *(animal protein)* with lightly steamed or sau-téed vegetables *(neutral)*
- Quinoa pasta *(starch)* with marinara *(neutral)* and shaved Manchego cheese *(animal protein)*, fresh basil, steamed vegetables *(neutral)* (technically not an ideal combination, but a better option than a gluten-containing wheat pasta with cow dairy Parmesan for those transitioning from a pasta-rich diet, and processed foods)
- Grilled chicken *(animal protein)* and teriyaki vegetable stir fry *(neutral)* (no rice)
- 3-whole-egg omelet *(animal protein)* with spinach *(neutral)*, tomatoes *(neutral)*, red bell pepper *(neutral)*, onion *(neutral)*, goat's milk feta cheese *(animal protein)*

- Sashimi *(animal protein)* with steamed vegetables *(neutral)* dipped into soy sauce *(neutral)*, preferably gluten-free (no rice)
- Brown rice bowl *(starch)* with steamed or grilled vegetables *(neutral)* and Mexican seasoning blend or drizzled with coconut aminos *(neutral)*

CHAPTER 5

Supplemental Practices

Supplements are not "one size fits all" nor are they a cure-all. If you're eating a poor diet, a handful of supplements are bound to stir up trouble when the root cause is not addressed. This particularly pertains to "colon cleanse" supplements that market "detox in a box" concepts, in addition to laxative products, which do not strengthen digestion and can create a lazy colon or dependency. If simply popping a pill were the solution, we would all be in picture-perfect health, no problem. With the appropriate diet plan and cleansing techniques however, the *right* supplements can help to heal and rejuvenate the skin more quickly.

Probiotics

Medicine disturbs the natural balance of healthy bacteria, or probiotics, in the gut. If you have ever been treated with antibiotics, you may have found your doctor recommending that you eat yogurt (or "acidophilus," a particular strain of probiotic) to counteract the medication.

Probiotics are beneficial ("good") microorganisms that help protect the body from harmful bacteria, strengthen immunity, enhance the functioning of the digestive system, and can be highly advantageous in eliminating yeast-related issues like candida. Because of their immune-boosting properties and support of the digestive tract, supplemental probiotics can help people with indigestion, irregularity, constipation, skin eruptions, and skin-related allergies, in addition to a variety of everyday imbalances, including low energy and mood swings.

A poor diet and any history of treatment with antibiotics is reason enough for anyone to start supplementing with probiotics today. Probiotics are safe for everyday use and are non-habit-forming. I believe that everyone, regardless of age, should supplement with probiotics, especially for a radiant and glowing complexion. That being said, just because a product contains probiotics does not necessarily make it beneficial, so don't head to the yogurt aisle just yet.

It is quite misleading to assume that yogurt will fill the void when circumstances have caused the body's beneficial probiotics to be depleted. As far as yogurt is concerned, the amounts of living microorganisms available are few and far between. Additionally, the sugar content in most yogurts far outweighs whatever "good" there may have been and can actually help feed toxic yeasts that create skin eruptions. Let's also not forget that yogurt is a dairy product and therefore acid-forming. As we now know, acid-forming foods offset our internal balance and wreak havoc on immunity and the skin. In addition to yogurt, other products that market themselves as containing probiotics like store-bought kefirs, kombucha, and probiotic "drinks" are in many ways just healthier alternatives to frozen yogurt or soda. Dairy-free alternatives to yogurt like coconut and almond yogurts can be fun transitional substitutes, but they should not serve as a replacement to high-quality sources of probiotic supplements. In fact, yogurt of any kind should not replace more alkaline and nutrient-dense breakfasts like fresh green juice and green smoothies.

In addition to using the supplements noted above, beneficial sources of probiotics include unpasteurized kimchi, cultured vegetables (sometimes called sauerkraut but other examples include: fermented cabbage, carrots, broccoli, onion), raw sauerkraut, homemade coconut kefir, and probiotic supplements in capsule or powder form. It is my recommendation that if candida overgrowth is suspected, one should avoid all fermented foods for the time being and take the supplement route.

Probiotic capsules are a convenient way to help these friendly bacteria colonize in the gut. They can be found in the refrigerated section of most health food stores or ordered directly online. It is important that the bottle specify "living organisms," as we want these active organisms to go to work digesting old wastes, reproducing, and strengthening the immune system.

The following are probiotic supplements I particularly like and have had a great deal of success with in my private practice:

- Raw Probiotics for Women by Garden of Life
- Raw Probiotics for Men by Garden of Life
- Dr. Ohhira's Probiotics

As for raw foods, I also love Rejuvenative Foods's kimchi and sauerkraut products, which can be located in your specialty health store in the refrigerated section.

Other Supplements

The skin acts as the backup for both the kidneys and liver. When either organ is suffering, the body will look to rid itself of excess toxicity through the skin. The following herbal supplements can aid in the detoxification process.

Scram by HealthForce Nutritionals: This formula is excellent for anyone who thinks they may have a candida-related disorder, has a history of antibiotic or prednisone use, skin-related disorders (especially acne), vaginal discomfort, suffers from itchy skin, hives, or easily gets rashes, struggles with weight-related problems, and/or someone who consumes, or has a history of consuming sugar, flour, processed foods, cooked fats and oils, an abundance of fruit, and/or alcohol (including wine). This supplement is not a substitute for a diet rich in these foods, nor does it countermeasure poor choices. In other words, Scram is not going be the solution without your desire to also make some lifestyle changes.

Scram works in addition to an alkaline diet and helps to manage cravings, improve digestion, strengthen immunity, and improve the quality of the skin by killing off the organisms that cause problems in the first place. Scram is strongly suggested for optimal results for the skin.

Para-Shield by Gaia: Para-Shield is also a beneficial formula and works similarly to Scram.

You can use these two supplements interchangeably, switching off between treatments over a period of time. There is no set time frame for how long you will want to take these supplements. It will be completely determined by your particular situation, including the level of your involvement in the program, how quick you are looking to see improvements, and your family health, wellness, and diet history (example: your genetic makeup and what food you grew up eating).

Digestive Enzymes by HealthForce Nutritionals: If your diet includes animal products and/or processed and heated foods, your digestion is not optimal. These foods do not contain their own food enzymes and therefore require the body to produce and use its own enzyme reserve, which diverts energy from the body. Taking digestive enzymes with meals can support the break down of food, enhance the rate at which nutrients are assimilated, and aid in a quicker evacuation to avoid the accumulation of waste and toxic byproducts. Once again, digestive enzymes do not replace a diet rich in foods with their own enzymes; these supplements are a non-habit forming method for improving waste removal. I recommend HealthForce for their superior, results-driven product line.

The following supplements can be taken alone or in combination with Scram and probiotic supplements. Each of these supplements is generally considered safe, but they are not intended for children or pregnant or lactating women. As with any supplement, you should always consult with your healthcare practitioner or nutritional consultant before making any significant dietary changes.

Milk thistle relieves congestion of the liver, spleen, and kidneys; it strengthens the liver's detoxification function.

Burdock root acts as a "blood purifier" by clearing toxins in the bloodstream to control skin inflammation.

Dandelion root is a mild diuretic that purifies the bloodstream and liver. It also stimulates the manufacture of bile.*

Garlic is considered "Russian penicillin" for its ability to effectively kill bacteria and parasites. Garlic is most beneficial consumed raw (as in chopped up in salads or atop freshly steamed veggies). If you do not tolerate the potency of garlic, it could be the way you are enjoying it. Coarsely chopping or thinly slicing garlic on a mandoline gives it an almost sweet flavor, while pulverizing or crushing garlic will emphasize its intensity. The more the cell walls of a garlic clove are damaged, the harsher the flavor will be. This has to do with the release of stored enzymes reacting with oxygen.

Note: Bile is an alkaline fluid that is stored in the gallbladder, but created and secreted by the liver in order to aid in the digestion and break down of fats. Bile also serves as a method for the removal of toxins, such as heavy metals, pharmaceuticals, carcinogens, and various chemicals the body comes in contact with. Without bile, the small intestine is unable to properly utilize fats or fat-soluble vitamins and can cause a toxic backup.

Deep Tissue Cleansing via Colon Hydrotherapy

The body functions as one unified organism, and the colon is an integral piece of this equation. The food (and drink) we choose to nourish our bodies with becomes the body's main source of fuel and energy. Unfit foods create inflammation and leave behind toxic residues and stagnant (or unmoving) waste matter for the body to rid itself of. When not efficiently eliminated, this waste is then stored in the intestinal tissue along with trapped gas from incomplete digestion and the fermented foods.

When the bowel becomes overloaded with an accumulation of impacted waste, gas, and toxins, it adds to the stress already on the organs and offsets the body's normal functioning. Toxins that cannot be eliminated through the bowels are released in the form of acne, asthma, dermatitis, colds, headaches, fever, anxiety, depression, and abnormal organ function. These "setbacks" are the body's mechanism for coping with and relieving itself of stress.

Alkaline foods awaken dormant toxins in an attempt to cleanse the body of these toxic stressors, hence the term "detox." As toxins are awakened by naturally cleansing foods, the need to remove these toxins efficiently becomes more essential to rapid improvements in health and a youthful radiance. In other words, once you have collected the garbage, it does no good to leave it out where the decay and smell can permeate the cleaner, newer house.

Due to our Westernized diet that is high in processed, artificial, and mass-produced foods, this waste is never completely eliminated from the body. Eating a cleansing diet is only part of the story, as we want to bring detrimental toxins to the surface so that they can be effectively removed. The idea of colon hydrotherapy (also referred to as colonic irrigation, colonics, or deep-tissue cleansing) is to remove the accumulation of impacted feces (old matter), waste, gas, and nonspecific toxins from within the colon tissue.

GRAVITY COLONICS

One method of aiding your body in ridding these toxins is gravity colonics. A gravity colonic works by cleansing the large intestine (colon) with warm (or cool) water that enters and simultaneously exits the body through a tube. During a gravity colonic, a 5-gallon tank of water is suspended above the body and refilled several times throughout the treatment. Water is carried through to the colon via the rectum, hydrating the tissue and allowing for a continuous exit of waste and toxins through thick tubing. A trained therapist works the abdomen, as they manually pump (or pulse) the water, which in turn activates the intestinal muscles to contract and relax, pushing out waste—a function called peristalsis. Just as any muscle will weaken without continuous use, the muscles that are part of the digestive tract become weak without "practice" in those more prone to constipation and thus digestion drastically slows as we age. A gravity colonic activates these muscles and helps it to work more effectively on a regular basis.

Colonics increase the rate at which the body can eliminate toxins and recover from acidity and disease. By increasing the rate at which waste is eliminated, stress is reduced from within. The cleansing of the colon is thus an incredible way to encourage the regeneration of cells throughout the body and skin. After a blockage of waste is removed during your first gravity colonic, you are likely to feel revitalized and lighter, and radiate a pleasant glow.

The amount needed is based on the individual and the rate at which detoxification is taking place. Remember: It took us years to accumulate this waste, we cannot expect it to all go out in one garbage bag, nor should we expect that a one-time renovation be enough.

For colon hydrotherapists in your area, contact the Helen Wood Institute for a directory of their graduates, trained and certified by Helen Wood, or visit www.detoxtheworld.com for a directory of therapists that have been recommended by some of my peers around the world.

If you are hesitant to try colon hydrotherapy, or there is not a therapist in your area, you may seek benefit by using a Cara Enema kit. Follow the instructions on the kit instruction. Note: An enema kit will not have the same "reach" as a colonic, nor will encourage peristalsis. That being said, it can be beneficial in loosening up and helping the body to remove some of the blockage occurring at that very last stretch of the colon.

WHAT COLONICS ARE NOT

- A counterbalance for a poor diet.
- A sole means of weight loss.
- An efficient cleansing method unless accompanied by a diet high in plant foods, which help to sweep food from the intestines to the colon.

A NOTE FOR THE LEERY

Deep-tissue cleansing from gravity colonics will produce profound results. Without some form of efficient cleansing, the results will be slower or plateau when the skin is the major concern, or the issue is severe.

For those who are uncomfortable with the idea of colonics, it is okay to ease into this lifestyle without it. You will certainly see great improvement when cleansing the body with good foods and juices.

It is very important to note that when we "awaken" a lifetime of stored "garbage" (impure material that has been causing the unwanted side effects of acne, and so on), we do not want to give it the opportunity to be reabsorbed into the bloodstream or cause further distress. It is for this reason that we must tread lightly and not rush into any "detox" too quickly, especially when colonics are not being administered.

One should only see a trained colon-hydrotherapist. The therapist should be in the room at all times. Be sure to discuss your medical history and conditions with your doctor and therapist prior to treatment. Always be sure to consult your medical advisor before considering a new lifestyle change or treatment.

Part II

CLEAR SKIN DETOX DIET

CHAPTER 6

Your New Diet Lifestyle for a Glowing Complexion

Goals Recap for All Diet Levels

Choosing foods that nourish and detoxify the skin for a clear complexion, youthful glow, and an overall radiant appearance is not about eating perfectly or making every dietary and lifestyle change overnight. Eating for beautiful skin is about making educated and conscious decisions that nourish your whole body, wherever you might be on your journey. The following goals will help you to make significant changes one step at a time, without feeling overwhelmed. Begin with goal number one, and challenge yourself to build from there.

Goal 1: Choose the foods that nourish.

This means choosing wholesome and natural plant foods that come from Mother Nature, instead of marketed "low-calorie" and "reduced-fat" items. The closest to "natural" we can get is to choose foods that grow from trees, vines, and the ground. The moment a food makes its way into a box or package, it has been processed to some degree. Foods that have long shelf lives are not generally as rich in vitamins, minerals, and enzymes as foods with shorter shelf lives. For instance, a sweet potato is more nutritious than a sweet potato chip, which has been baked in oils and salted.

- Steer clear of fast food, highly processed food, and frozen TV dinners.
- If a food has more than four ingredients in it, and they are items other than herbs, spices, and whole foods such as organic ground corn, look for alternatives so that you can reduce and eliminate this from your diet.
- Eliminate milk and dairy products (with the exception of organic butter for flavor and sautéing and goat and sheep's milk cheeses).
- Eliminate soy products with the exception of a minimal amount of soy sauce (preferably use gluten-free tamari, Bragg's Liquid Aminos, or ideally coconut aminos) and organic fermented miso.
- Eliminate sodas, both diet and regular.
- Reduce and eventually eliminate carbonated beverages. Carbonated beverages disrupt digestion and create gas, trapping waste in the intestinal tract.
- Reduce stimulants like caffeine, which also often serve in place of more alkaline meals. Instead, begin the morning with something more nutrient-dense and alkaline such as a juice and/or a smoothie.
- Make greens and vegetables the focal point of every meal. If you love cheese, use it as a flavor instead of the meal itself. You will find you have much more energy and more beautiful skin as a result. For instance, a big bowl of freshly steamed broccoli with your favorite marinara or 1

tablespoon of organic butter and a sprinkling of Manchego sheep's milk cheese following a salad is perfectly fine.

Goal #2: Always eat something raw before eating something cooked.

- Start every meal with a *living* green, like "a dinner salad."
- Prepare. If you know you are going to be grabbing lunch out with your coworkers, show up to work with a baggy of celery sticks, raw carrots, or raw sweet potato slices to enjoy prior to a questionable meal.

Goal #3: Enjoy foods in the right combinations.

- Eat fruit alone or leave it at home.
- The only time fruit can be combined with vegetables is in the form of a green juice, in which the fiber is removed and thus does not require digestion, and in a green smoothie. A green smoothie is a blend of leafy greens, plant-based vegetables, minimal fruit for sweetness, and water. The act of blending helps to predigest these foods. Juices and smoothies should be consumed on an empty stomach and never eaten with a meal.
- It is not advisable to add seeds, nuts, or denser foods with fruits in a smoothie. Just because something looks appealing on paper does not mean the body can quickly digest and assimilate the nutrients as so. In other words, although apples are a great source of fiber, and contain a special phytonutrient that helps to cleanse our blood, it does not make it more powerful and nutritious to combine apples with another nutrient-dense food with strong anti-inflammatory benefits like flax seeds or their oils. Apples and seeds do not digest well together.
- Separate starches from proteins.

- Leave at least three to four hours between meals before switching to a different category of foods, unless it is an all-fruit meal.
- Refrain from drinking water with meals, as it will dilute digestive enzymes.
- Enjoy 8 to 24 ounces of water in the morning before consuming anything else. This will keep your cells hydrated.

Goal #4: Have fun.
- Experiment in the kitchen.
- Enjoy your favorite flavors.
- Delight in having the knowledge you need to be your most beautiful and radiant self.

Determine Your Diet Plan

The above pointers will help you get started. Use the charts in this book, such as "Build a Better Salad" (page 79) in order to create satisfying, nutrient-dense, and well-combined meals. Use the "Food Combining" chart (page 194) to help make better combinations daily for enhanced digestion and assimilation of nutrients. Use the "General Grocery Shopping List" (page 200) as a reference when shopping for your favorite items and the "Best Options When Dining Out" chart (page 198) to assist you in making the smartest choices when preparing and choosing from common menu items.

The following meal plans, New Leaf Beauty (page 125), New Light Beauty (page 127), and Glow Lifestyle (page 129) are separated based on your current diet's inclusion of meat, cheese, and vegetables. These are lifestyle plans that have more specific recipes to give you an idea for several days of unique meals, but you are certainly not limited to these dishes. Use the "Food Combining" chart (page 194) and "Build a Better Salad" chart (page 79) to construct a plan based on your preferences.

New Leaf Beauty

Follow this plan if you're ready to turn over a new leaf and discover the beautiful skin you desire but you would like to keep meat in your diet. The menu is primarily plant-based and predominately alkaline but includes cheese, eggs, and fish. Other high-quality meat products can be used in place of fish. Keep consumption of eggs, fish, and other animal-based proteins for dinner. Light consumption of cheese for lunch is fine.

Allow this plan to give you an idea of how your day should go. Or use the "Food Combining" chart on page 194 and additional diagrams to make your own!

New Leaf Beauty Daily Routine

Morning	**Hydrate**: Upon waking, drink at least 8 ounces of pure spring water to hydrate your cells.
	Detoxify: Heat 4 to 6 ounces of water on the stovetop. Halve one lemon and squeeze its juice into a mug. Add water and enjoy.
	Supplement: Start with a multivitamin and probiotics. I recommend Garden of Life brand for their superior plant-based products.
	Infuse: When hungry, enjoy 16 to 32 ounces of (ideally) freshly pressed green vegetable juice. In many cases, it is acceptable to use an apple to sweeten. If you wish to start your morning with a green smoothie instead of, or in addition to, you may do so here.
Evening	**Hydrate**: Wind down after dinner with herbal tea if you're used to "snacking." Sweeten with stevia, if needed, and ¼ cup of almond milk.
	Supplement: Take additional supplements before bedtime: Scram by HealthForce and Oil of Oregano by Gaia.

New Leaf Beauty Recipe Options

Juices	Sunshine Lemonade (page 143)
	Bunny Love (page 143)
	Beauty Tonic (page 144)
Smoothies	Snow White (page 147)
	Radiant Greens (page 147)
Lunch	Glow Detox Kale Salad (page 154)
	Mediterranean Salad (page 150)
	Country Club Salad (page 156)
Sides *(interchangeable based on combination of entrée)*	*Add these to your salads or serve them in addition to greens.*
	Miso-Glazed Eggplant (page 160)
	Curried Sweet Potatoes (page 159)
	Steamed or grilled vegetables
Dinner	Baked Eggplant Rollatini with Roasted Red Pepper Filling (page 171)
	Spicy Puttanesca Sauce (page 166) with zucchini noodles
	Pan-Seared Ahi Tuna Teriyaki (page 169)
	Greek Omelet (page 175)
Sides *(interchangeable based on combination of entrée)*	Roasted Golden Beets and Fennel in Honey-Mustard Glaze (page 161)
	Bunless Cheese "Burger" (page 168)
	Steamed or grilled vegetables
Dessert	Avoid eating fruit after dinner, and instead enjoy 3 to 4 squares of organic dark chocolate (70% cacao and above) if needed.

New Light Beauty

If you are an experienced dieter or an avid exerciser and you are now ready to view your health in a new light, follow this plan to get the whole package. The plan is mostly plant-based and predominately alkaline but includes cheese and eggs. There is not a focus on grains or soy, as is usual for a vegetarian-oriented lifestyle. Keep consumption of eggs to dinner. Light consumption of cheese for lunch is fine, but ideally we are saving all animal proteins for our dinner meals.

Allow this plan to give you an idea of how your day should go. Or use the "Food Combining" chart on page 194 and additional diagrams to make your own!

New Light Beauty Daily Routine

Morning	**Hydrate**: Upon waking, drink at least 8 ounces of pure spring water to hydrate your cells.
	Detoxify: Heat 4 to 6 ounces of water on the stovetop. Halve one lemon and squeeze its juice into a mug. Add water and enjoy.
	Supplement: Start with a multivitamin and probiotics. I recommend Garden of Life brand for their superior plant-based products.
	Infuse: When hungry, enjoy 16 to 32 ounces of (ideally) freshly pressed green vegetable juice. In many cases, it is acceptable to use an apple to sweeten. If you wish to start your morning with a green smoothie instead of, or in addition to, you may do so here.
Evening	**Hydrate**: Wind down after dinner with herbal tea if you're used to "snacking." Sweeten with stevia, if needed, and ¼ cup of almond milk.
	Supplement: Take additional supplements before bedtime: Scram by HealthForce and Oil of Oregano by Gaia.

New Light Beauty Recipe Options

Juices	Sunshine Lemonade (page 143)
	Bunny Love (page 143)
	Beauty Tonic (page 144)
Smoothies	Snow White (page 147)
	Radiant Greens (page 147)
Lunch	Glow Detox Kale Salad (page 154)
	Mediterranean Salad (page 150)
	Country Club Salad (page 156)
Sides *(interchangeable based on combination of entrée)*	*Add these to your salads or serve them in addition to greens.*
	Portabella Mushroom Steaks (page 170)
	Curried Sweet Potatoes (page 159)
	Simple Nori Burrito (page 176)
Dinner	Baked Eggplant Rollatini with Roasted Red Pepper Filling (page 171)
	Creamy Quick Kelp Noodles (page 172)
	Almond-Crusted Eggplant (page 175)
	3 whole-egg omelet with spinach, diced tomatoes, and onion
Sides *(interchangeable based on combination of entrée)*	Seasoned Shiitake Mushrooms (page 159)
	Roasted Cauliflower (page 162)
	Steamed vegetables
Dessert	Avoid eating fruit after dinner, and instead enjoy 3 to 4 squares of organic dark chocolate (70% cacao and above) if needed.

Glow Lifestyle

You have been enjoying a relatively balanced and otherwise clean and healthful diet and you are ready to put on the finishing touches. Here you are challenged to reevaluate your beliefs and unveil your most beautiful and radiant skin. This plan focuses primarily on plant-based options and eliminates all animal products. There is not a focus on grains or soy, as is usual for an animal-free lifestyle. If you wish to enjoy a gluten-free grain, do so for dinner.

Allow this plan to give you an idea of how your day should go. Or use the "Food Combining" chart on page 194 and additional diagrams to make your own!

Glow Lifestyle Daily Routine

Morning	**Hydrate**: Upon waking, drink at least 8 ounces of pure spring water to hydrate your cells.
	Detoxify: Heat 4 to 6 ounces of water on the stovetop. Halve one lemon and squeeze its juice into a mug. Add water and enjoy.
	Supplement: Start with a multivitamin and probiotics. I recommend Garden of Life brand for their superior plant-based products.
	Infuse: When hungry, enjoy 16 to 32 ounces of (ideally) freshly pressed green vegetable juice. In many cases, it is acceptable to use an apple to sweeten. If you wish to start your morning with a green smoothie instead of, or in addition to, you may do so here.
Evening	**Hydrate**: Wind down after dinner with herbal tea if you're used to "snacking." Sweeten with stevia, if needed, and ¼ cup of almond milk.
	Supplement: Take additional supplements before bedtime: Scram by HealthForce and Oil of Oregano by Gaia.

Glow Lifestyle Recipe Options

Juices	Sunshine Lemonade (page 143)
	Bunny Love (page 143)
	Beauty Tonic (page 144)
Smoothies	Snow White (page 147)
	Radiant Greens (page 147)
Lunch	Glow Detox Kale Salad (page 154)
	Mediterranean Salad (page 150)
	Country Club Salad (page 156)
Sides *(interchangeable based on combination of entrée)*	*Add these to your salads or serve them in addition to greens.*
	Portabella Mushroom Steaks (page 170)
	Curried Sweet Potatoes (page 159)
	Simple Nori Burrito (page 176)
Dinner	Baked Eggplant Rollatini with Roasted Red Pepper Filling (page 171)
	Creamy Quick Kelp Noodles (page 172)
	Almond-Crusted Eggplant (page 175)
Sides *(interchangeable based on combination of entrée)*	Seasoned Shiitake Mushrooms (page 159)
	Roasted Cauliflower (page 162)
	Steamed vegetables
Dessert	Avoid eating fruit after dinner, and instead enjoy 3 to 4 squares of organic dark chocolate (70% cacao and above) if needed.

Basic Guidelines

Regardless of which plan you're following, use these "Basic Guidelines" as a reminder and outline for living this lifestyle every day. This is a journey. Be at peace knowing you are on your way to beautiful skin, and integrate better eating habits gradually, one day at a time. The more greens you can add to your diet, the fewer processed and acid-forming foods you will crave. It is magical!

AVOID

- Soda: diet and regular
- Carbonated beverages
- Artificial sweeteners (except stevia)
- Protein shakes, bars, and supplements
- All juices that are not considered fresh and raw (not heated or flash-pasteurized)
- Red meat, especially non-organically raised animals or animals that are not grass-fed
- Deli meats
- Imitation meats (tofu)
- Soy milk, foods containing soy (with the exception of soy lecithin, found in most processed foods)
- Refined sugar, refined starches, and agave
- Table salt
- Dairy (exceptions: raw goat/raw sheep)
- Fried foods
- Microwaved foods
- Popcorn
- Alcohol (except wine—vodka is harsh on the liver but preferred over beer and rums)
- Mainstream salad dressings and balsamic vinegars (always rinse olives to avoid excess salt and vinegars)

HIGHLIGHTS

- Focus on hydrating the cells with water first thing in the morning, prior to consumption of anything else
- Continue introducing the body to alkalizing vitamins, minerals, and raw enzymes in the morning via freshly pressed vegetable juice, and/or a green smoothie
- Focus on eating something "light" and raw prior to consuming something cooked
- Practice food combining: which means keeping starches separate from animal proteins at every meal, and keeping nuts, seeds, and dried fruit at least three to four hours separate from meals that contain either starches or animal proteins
- Restrict meat consumption to dinner (high-quality fish is preferred)
- Focus on enjoying a vegetarian dinner at least three times a week
- Agave is a well-marketed sugar, which does not do the body good. However, there is organic agave-sweetened ketchup that is a good alternative to traditional condiments

NEUTRAL FOODS

- Lemon/lime juice
- Olive oil
- Organic real butter
- Celtic sea salt
- Minimal organic dark chocolate
- Leafy greens and sea veggies
- Raw low-starch vegetables (carrots, peppers—all except green, which are gassy—cucumbers, cherry tomatoes)
- Low-starch steamed vegetables (broccoli, zucchini—both yellow and green)

- Stevia
- Raw honey
- B grade maple syrup

THE BREAKFAST ESSENTIALS: (ONLY TO BE CONSUMED ON AN EMPTY STOMACH)

Taking in juice first thing on an empty stomach allows the body to assimilate and absorb nutrients the most rapidly, cleansing the blood, and energizing your body for take off, healing, and cell regeneration. It is to be consumed after hydrating with water and throughout the morning (before any solid food). It acts to nourish the body quickly because it requires virtually no digestion and is chockfull of raw vitamins, minerals, oxygen, water, and vegetable sugar. Hallelujah! Following are two basic recipes that you can come back to anytime.

Go-To Juice Recipe

You can get this at a smoothie place.

10 large organic carrots (or 1 to 2 small apples)
1 medium beet (or celery if using apple)
1 small handful organic parsley leaves and stems
½ organic cucumber
2 handfuls organic spinach + other favorite greens

If fresh vegetable juices are not realistic for you at the moment, we will focus on making green smoothies your "rock star."

Ideally, one would consume fresh juice prior to incorporating smoothies. A smoothie is a combination of "predigested" fruits and vegetables. A smoothie contains the plant cellulose, or fiber from the plant, which makes us feel full longer and delays absorption. This smoothie is a GREAT way to start.

Go-To Green Smoothie

　　1½ ripe (freckled) bananas (frozen optional)
　　½ organic large green apple
　　1½ cups pure spring water
　　2 handfuls organic spinach
　　1 small handful parsley leaves and stems
　　1 small handful mint leaves and stems
　　1 squirt fresh lemon juice (optional)
　　sprinkle of cinnamon (optional)

Note: If you do not like parsley, try cilantro.

CHAPTER 7

Frequently Asked Questions

Q. *What about balsamic vinegar and balsamic vinaigrettes?*
A. Balsamic vinegar is highly acid-forming, offsets pH, and feeds candida. If you are having a terrible time moving away from Caesar, ranch, low-fat, and/or other mass-marketed dressings, then a table-spoon or less of balsamic is OK on occasion, but it is *not* a healthy dressing to use for beautiful skin.

Raw apple cider vinegar is the only exception to the "no vinegar" rule and can be used in moderate amounts as a dressing. Because it is unpasteurized and fermented, apple cider vinegar, with no added ingredients or sugars (unlike kombucha), will ideally still contain beneficial properties. That being said, if you notice any skin irritation, persisting or new blemishes, or you feel any discomfort or indigestion consuming apple cider vinegar, hold off on consuming any vinegars until you can better assess your body's reaction.

Q. *But our ancestors ate grains. How can whole grains not be good for us?*
A. Have you noticed the amount of food products, even desserts, that advertise their new whole-grain ingredients? This is very misleading. Wheat is very acid-forming. Our ancestors enjoyed pure,

unprocessed, living grains grown in nutrient-dense soils. The bread and similar whole-grain products of today are no match for those of yesteryear. They are mass cultivated in overworked soil, depleted of nutrients, often covered in chemical fertilizers, and then processed and heated to high temperatures. There is nothing living or nutritious about these foods, save perhaps their fiber content (which leads to constipation because it's devoid of living enzymes). Grain products are then fortified (i.e., synthetic vitamins and minerals are added) to seem "healthy."

Alternatives to "whole grains": The most alkaline grains are amaranth, buckwheat, millet, and quinoa. Spelt and Kamut are slightly more acid-forming. Baked organic corn and corn tortillas can also be used as an occasional substitute for dipping into guacamole or hummus and Tex Mex.

Q. *What about rice?*
A. My answer is similar to the above: most rice is processed, bleached, and treated. On top of that, have you ever noticed how sticky rice becomes after cooking? Imagine how much of an indigestible and pasty nightmare it becomes for the digestive system. Constipation! If you do eat rice, make sure it is a wild or a brown rice, and combine it properly with starches. Be sure to start your meal with a delicious leafy green salad. To facilitate digestion, I do not recommend combining rice with beans. Rice should be eaten with greens and vegetables, not animal products, nuts, seeds, or dried fruit.

Q. *What about gluten-free?*
A. "Gluten-free" products are a marketer's dream. The term seems to be slapped on innumerable products these days—even ones that should not need a stamp (like marinara sauce, mustard, or ketchup, for instance).

So what is gluten? Gluten is the protein found in wheat and it is highly acid-forming in our bodies. Gluten is difficult to digest, void of nutrients, and highly inflammatory, and it can lead to an assortment of bodily discomforts, including but not limited to, skin disorders, digestive difficulty, arthritis, and weight gain.

Many, although not all, "gluten-free" products like pasta, bread, muffins, and desserts, among others, are made with rice and generally have additives with long names and synthetic fillers to bridge the gap or invite flavor where it is lacking. While these products may bring temporary relief to those who are very noticeably sensitive to "gluten," they only invite other problems. Rice is highly constipating! It slows digestion and therefore creates skin problems. Additionally, many of these "gluten-free" products might be loaded with sugars and fats to compensate for a lack of gluten, flavor, and texture.

The best alternatives to rice and mass-marketed "gluten-free" products are "low-to-no gluten" sprouted grains like millet and quinoa. Gluten-free products made with amaranth, buckwheat, millet, quinoa, and corn are perfectly acceptable. Treat them as starches and keep them apart from animal proteins, nuts, seeds, and dried fruit as well as fruits!

Q. *What about an all-raw diet?*
A. When I see dieters who have gone entirely raw, I am concerned about a few things. First of all, there is the worry that they are eating too many nut and seed products. These foods are dense and difficult to digest, especially when eaten in quantities of more than ¼ cup or when they are wrongly combined. Then there is the concern that, although raw, there is too much sugar from an abundance of fruits and denser dried fruits. I am also worried about how people on a raw diet are combining the foods they are eating. For example, nuts and avocados, though both raw, do not combine well and

will slow digestion. Finally, there is a concern that some veggies like the cruciferous broccoli, cauliflower, and Brussels sprouts do not digest well when they are completely raw. Although someone may have great success at first with an "all-raw" diet, skin, energy, and weight-loss plateaus usually become an issue later on.

Q. *I am so full of energy that I'm having trouble sleeping. How many hours of sleep do I need?*

A. There's no doubt that this lifestyle increases energy. In fact, you may have so much energy you feel like you can keep on going and going and going. But sleeping is crucial to overall health and a beautiful complexion. Sleep is when the body has the time to destress and focus on detoxifying. Seven to nine hours is an ideal amount of sleep. Trouble sleeping when on a detox plan is not uncommon during the initial days. Toxins that have been "awakened" and not yet eliminated can be a cause. Colon hydrotherapy can solve this. Plant-based magnesium can also help to naturally relax the body and increase bowel movements; look for it in the supplement section of your health food store.

Q. *Is it true that you should stop eating before 8:00 pm? How would this affect my skin?*

A. This rule is not in place because some magical fairy pulls the trigger and stops metabolism at a certain time. Eating closer to bedtime slows digestion and allows stomach acids to creep back into your esophagus. This creates acid reflux, discomfort, and indigestion. Digestion, assimilation of nutrients, and elimination of waste are key to beautiful skin. Indigestion and stomach reflux is not. Additionally, when the body is at rest, its goal is to restore and regenerate. When it is given food before bedtime, energy will be diverted to digestion instead of focusing on the key benefits of sleep: detoxification, restoration, rejuvenation, and the regeneration of cells.

For best digestion and therefore a radiant complexion, your last meal of the day should be eaten three to four hours before hitting the sheets.

Q. *How much water do I need?*
A. Drinking water with meals dilutes digestive enzymes. Ideally, beverages should not be consumed with food for optimal digestion. When your diet is rich in vegetables (and not overloaded with salt), that hydrating produce will provide the body with beneficial H_2O. That being said, the body will require different amounts of water depending on activity level and temperature. During the hot summer (or during more rigorous exercise), for instance, the body sweats more and therefore requires hydration. Listen to your body. Upon waking, and/or before anything else is consumed, hydrate your body with pure, filtered or bottled drinking water. Do not force yourself to drink water, as is often suggested in different diet programs. This is not beneficial and only slows digestion. Water, freshly pressed vegetable juices, and to a lesser extent, moderate amounts of unpasteurized, raw coconut water from a young Thai coconut, is all the liquid the body requires for hydration. When you are drinking coffees, non-herbal teas, and cacao, beverages that act as diuretics and deplete the body of water, or even taking medication that dehydrates the body, you will need more water to offset this action.

Q. *But I need coffee. When can I have my coffee?*
A. Coffee and non-herbal teas are acid-forming. They are also stimulants and do not provide authentic or lasting energy. You will find that when digestion is improved and juice is consumed, your energy levels will skyrocket. If you still feel that you need coffee or just like the taste, enjoy it 30 minutes before or 30 minutes after your freshly pressed vegetable juice.

It's fine if you love coffee! Coffee is not *bad* to enjoy, so do not feel *bad* doing so. If you are making other beneficial changes to your diet, the coffee should be the least of your worries. Limit yourself to one cup per day. Just do yourself a favor and *enjoy* the coffee. Thinking bad thoughts about food is not beneficial either.

• • • •

BUT WHAT ABOUT ALCOHOL AND SMOKING?

It should go without saying that certain things are not beneficial to the body or skin.

Drinking Alcohol

Regardless of what you hear about the benefits of wine, wine is dehydrating, intoxicating, high in sugar, and though initially a sedative, disrupts deep, restorative sleep. That being said, drinking is a social activity and it can be enjoyed in this lifestyle. The "best" alcoholic beverage is wine and is fine in moderation. Moderation is a broad term, but for our purposes, many of my clients can have one to two glasses of wine on the weekends and a glass of wine on a week night, should they desire it instead of a piece of bread or slice of pizza. A glass of wine is fine with dinner when dinner is a well-combined vegetable dish, if it is instead of a burger or a pasta covered with cheese. I find that clients are much more amenable to eating a nutrient-dense dinner and feel less restricted if they can also have a glass of wine.

If you have severe acne or skin discomforts, alcohol should be eliminated from your diet until the healthy bacteria is restored and your body's pH is in balance. If you are going to be enjoying a cocktail, vodka is the better option among common liquors. Though harsher on the liver than wine, it is typically less processed than other hard liquors. It is best consumed with water and fresh lemon and/or lime juice. Avoid mixers and diet and regular sodas. Beer is yeast-forming, disrupts digestion, and has no place in a healthy diet or skin care regimen. It causes bloating and stimulates the growth of candida.

Smoking

Not only does it completely infect the lungs, cause cancer, and penetrate the entire body with noxious toxins (nicotine, carbon monoxide, cadmium, etc.), smoking increases free radical formation, which causes rapid aging of the skin. Want to reverse aging and improve skin tone, elasticity, and complexion? DON'T SMOKE.

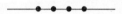

CHAPTER 8

Glow Detox Recipes

Juices

Unless otherwise noted, fruits and vegetables do not need to be peeled, although rinsing is necessary. Organic is always preferred, especially when juicing and drinking produce. When we juice or blend our greens and fruits, we are enabling easier and quicker absorption of their nutrients—but also their pesticides. While it is not always required that your produce is organic, try to at least stick to the Dirty Dozen, and especially aim to use organic produce when juicing. For more information about what produce should be purchased organic, and when it is OK to purchase non-organic items, refer to the "Clean Fifteen" and "Dirty Dozen" mentioned earlier in this book.

Rebalance

This juice is exceptional for enhancing digestion and offers an immediate boost of energy.

Combines with: Juice is best consumed alone, for breakfast, and not combined with other foods.

Yield: 1 serving

2½ pounds carrots
½ large beet
½ inch gingerroot
¼ bunch cilantro

Pass each ingredient through your juicer, alternating leafy greens between more solid vegetables to facilitate juicing. For instance, you may wish to put ginger, then cilantro, followed by carrots and beets through your juicer, in that order.

Sunshine Lemonade

Hydrating, refreshing, and alkalizing, this juice is like sipping on sunshine.

Combines with: Juice is best consumed alone, for breakfast, and not combined with other foods.

Yield: 1 serving

2 small pears or small Fuji apples
½ lemon, with peel
¼ bunch kale (2 to 4 stems)
1 cup packed spinach (1 large handful)
2 stalks celery
½ cucumber, with skin

Pass each ingredient through your juicer in the order shown.

Bunny Love

A quick energy boost, this juice is high in vitamins A and C and calcium.

Combines with: Juice is best consumed alone, for breakfast, and not combined with other foods.

Yield: 1 serving

2½ pounds carrots, rinsed but unpeeled
2 handfuls spinach leaves

Pass each ingredient through your juicer, alternating between carrots and spinach.

Carrot Ginger

Wonderful for digestion, carrot juice and ginger help to heal inflammation and support metabolism.

Combines with: Juice is best consumed alone, for breakfast, and not combined with other foods, however, juice from root vegetables (carrot, beet, ginger) without the addition of quickly fermenting juices from fruits or greens, can be consumed later on throughout your day as a snack.

Yield: 1 serving

2½ pounds carrots
½ inch gingerroot, unpeeled

Pass each ingredient through your juicer, alternating between carrots and ginger.

Beauty Tonic

This tart, alkaline juice works to detoxify, hydrate, and tighten the skin.

Combines with: Juice is best consumed alone, for breakfast, and not combined with other foods.

Yield: 1 serving

1 whole cucumber, unpeeled
¼ bunch parsley
1 large Granny Smith apple
1 handful spinach

Pass each ingredient through your juicer alternating the leafy greens between the solid apple and cucumber.

Green is Queen

This highly alkalizing juice is a blend of beautifying vitamins, minerals, enzymes, and H$_2$O.

Combines with: Juice is best consumed alone, for breakfast, and not combined with other foods.

Yield: 1 serving

   1 medium to large whole cucumber, with skin
   ¼ bunch parsley
   3 stalks celery
   1 large head romaine
   ½ medium lemon (optional)

Pass each ingredient through your juicer, alternating parsley between solid vegetables.

Beauty Cocktail

This juice is every bit as fun as it is beautifying.

Combines with: Juice is best consumed alone, for breakfast, and not combined with other foods.

Yield: 1 serving

   ½ large lime, peeled if not organic
   1 medium orange, peeled
   5 stalks celery
   1 large handful spinach
   1 head romaine or ½ large cucumber

Pass each ingredient through your juicer alternating between ingredients.

Pumpkin Milk

Pumpkin milk is made with a juicer, not a blender, but it has a milky consistency.

Combines with: Juice is best consumed alone, for breakfast, and not combined with other foods.

Yield: 1 serving

> 1 large sweet potato
> 5 stalks celery
> 1 inch burdock root
> ½ inch gingerroot, unpeeled
> 1 teaspoon ground cinnamon
> 1 drop liquid vanilla stevia (optional)

Pass the first 4 ingredients through a juicer. Whisk in the cinnamon. Add the stevia, if using.

Smoothies

Green smoothies are a delicious way to drink your greens for breakfast and begin the day with an abundance of nutrients but also fiber. Green smoothies are best enjoyed as a breakfast meal, and not with other foods, for increased nutrient absorption and enhanced digestion. Although we talk about enjoying fruits alone, green smoothies are an exception to the rule because the blending process actually helps to "pre-digest" the fruit and greens and break down the fibers. However, it is not OK to add in nuts or seeds. I would also advise against protein powders and milks. The goal of the smoothie is to quickly nourish, and denser foods will slow down that process. In other words, more is not always better.

When making smoothies with a standard low-speed blender, it can be helpful to begin with frozen fruit and water, blending until smooth, and then adding in your greens, blending again until a smooth consistency is achieved. When using a high-powered blender like the Vitamix or Blendtec, order will not matter.

Radiant Greens

Combines with: Smoothies are best consumed alone, for breakfast, and should not be combined with other foods. The blending of the greens with quick-digesting fruit helps our body more rapidly digest and break down the nutrients.

Yield: 1 serving

> 1½ large ripe bananas, peeled and frozen
> 1½ cups water
> 2 cups organic spinach or kale leaves
> ½ bunch fresh parsley, including stems
> ½ cup fresh or frozen organic blueberries
> ¼ cup chopped fennel bulb (or ¼ large fennel bulb, chopped)

In a high-speed blender, combine the bananas, water, and spinach or kale. Blend until the bananas are smooth and then add the remaining ingredients. Blend until smooth. Serve cold.

Snow White

Combines with: Smoothies are best consumed alone, for breakfast, and should not be combined with other foods. The blending of the greens with quick-digesting fruit helps our body more rapidly digest and break down the nutrients.

Yield: 1 serving

> 1 large ripe banana, peeled and frozen
> 1½ cups water
> 2 cups spinach
> 4 leaves romaine
> 1½ medium apples, Granny Smith or Fuji
> 1 teaspoon ground cinnamon

In a high-speed blender, combine the banana, water, and spinach. Blend until the bananas are smooth and then add the remaining ingredients. Blend until smooth. Serve cold.

Milks

"The Milky Way" Walnut Milk

A fantastic source of omega-3 fatty acids and antioxidants, the combination of walnuts and raw cacao will have you radiating beautiful skin and energy. Walnut milk can be enjoyed over ice, in place of milk in cereal, or in your coffee, tea, or hot cacao. Use as you would milk. When enjoyed alone, it is best chilled or lightly warmed in blender or on the stovetop.

Combines with: Neutral foods

Yield: about 4 cups

> 1 cup raw walnuts, soaked for 2 to 4 hours in water, then drained
> 4 cups filtered water
> 5 tablespoons raw cacao
> stevia or vanilla stevia, to taste

Blend the walnuts and pure water in a high-speed blender. Pour through a nut milk bag over a large bowl and then strain. Stir in the remaining ingredients or mix in your blender. Store in an airtight glass jar for up to 5 days in the refrigerator. Serve as you like.

Sunflower Seed Sunshine Milk

An excellent source of vitamin E, a free radical–fighting antioxidant, and the naturally calming mineral magnesium, this alkaline, mood-enhancing beverage will be having you feeling satiated, glowing, and young. Sunflower Seed Sunshine Milk can be enjoyed over ice, in place of milk in cereal, or in your coffee, tea, or hot cacao. Use as you would milk. When enjoyed alone, it is best chilled or lightly warmed in blender or on the stovetop.

Combines with: Neutral foods

Yield: about 4 cups

> 1 cup raw hulled sunflower seeds, soaked for 2 to 4 hours
> in water, then drained
> 4 cups pure water
> stevia or vanilla stevia, to taste

Blend the soaked sunflower seeds and pure water in a high-speed blender. Pour through a nut milk bag over a large bowl and then strain. Stir in the remaining ingredients or mix in your blender. Store in an airtight glass jar for up to 5 days in the refrigerator. Serve as you like.

Salads

Garlic Stir-Fried Snow Peas and Pea Greens

Combines with: Neutral foods

Yield: 2–4 servings

> 1 tablespoon water
> 2 tablespoons chopped garlic
> 2 tablespoons chopped gingerroot
> 2 cups snow peas, or snap peas, trimmed
> 2 cups pea sprouts, packed
> 1 cup frozen peas, thawed
> 1 tablespoon gluten-free low-sodium tamari

Heat a large skillet over high heat. Add the water, garlic, and ginger; cook, stirring, until fragrant, 10 to 15 seconds. Add the snow peas or snap peas and stir until they turn bright green and the garlic is just barely browning, about 1 minute. Stir in the pea sprouts, thawed peas, and tamari. Stir for another 30 seconds to 1 minute, allowing the pea sprouts to wilt. Transfer to a serving dish and enjoy!

Floral Spring Salad

Combines with: Neutral foods

Yield: 2–4 servings

 8 ounces baby greens

 3 ounces snow pea shoots, chopped

 1 medium cucumber, peeled, sliced into medallions

 1 cup artichoke hearts, halved

 1 cup yellow, purple, and orange carrots, sliced into medallions

 2 tablespoons diced red onion

 1 cup baby tomatoes, halved

 8 medium asparagus spears, peeled with a vegetable peeler into long, skinny slivers

 3 garlic cloves, shaved on a mandoline

 ½ cup fresh lemon juice

 1 teaspoon raw apple cider vinegar (optional)

 ⅛ teaspoon Celtic sea salt

 freshly ground black pepper

 ½ cup edible flowers

Mix together the first nine ingredients in a large bowl. Dress with lemon juice, vinegar, if using, salt, and pepper to taste. Plate salad on a serving dish, and then arrange edible flowers on top for décor.

Mediterranean Salad

Combines with: Neutral foods, Animal protein

Yield: 2–4 servings

 1 cup baby tomatoes, halved

 8 ounces baby romaine lettuce

 ¼ cup diced red onion

 2 cups artichoke hearts, coarsely chopped

 ½ cup Castelvetrano olives (mild green olives)

 1 tablespoon coarsely chopped or torn fresh basil

2 tablespoons raw apple cider vinegar

freshly ground black pepper

Toss the all ingredients in a large bowl and sprinkle with freshly ground black pepper to taste. To make this heartier, add ¾ cup freshly shredded raw sheep's or raw goat's milk cheese.

Coleslaw Salad

Serve this as a side dish for marinated barbecued mushrooms or enjoy it as a creamy salad.

Combines with: Starch

Yield: 1 salad or 4 side servings

1 head romaine lettuce, finely chopped

1 cup shredded carrots

1 cup shredded zucchini

½ large avocado, cubed

2 tablespoons Dijon Vinaigrette (page 157)

Combine all the ingredients in a large bowl and mix well.

Greek Cucumber Salad

Combines with: Animal protein

Yield: 2–4 servings

4 large English cucumbers, peeled and diced

⅛ teaspoon sea salt, plus more

1 cup pitted Cerignola olives, halved (large, mild green olives)

¼ cup diced raw goat's or sheep's cheese

½ cup diced red onion

¼ cup raw apple cider vinegar

2 tablespoons chopped fresh basil

⅛ teaspoon dried oregano

⅛ teaspoon dried thyme

Place the diced cucumbers in a colander and sprinkle with sea salt. Leave to drain for 20 minutes while you prep the other ingredients. Pat the cucumbers dry, absorbing the excess water, and combine with all the ingredients in a large bowl. Serve immediately, or allow flavors to marinate overnight in a covered container. Marinating will give the cucumbers more time to absorb the flavors, but in the case of overnight marinating, save the basil and cheese for when you're ready to serve, or the basil will brown.

Cooling Cucumber Salad

Combines with: Starch

Yield: 4–6 servings

> 4 large English cucumbers, peeled and thinly sliced into medallions
> ½ teaspoon pink Himalayan salt, divided
> 1 large avocado, cubed (optional)
> 1 cup thinly sliced shallots
> 2 large garlic cloves, thinly sliced on a mandoline
> ¼ cup raw apple cider vinegar
> 2 tablespoons chopped fresh dill
> 1 tablespoon chopped fresh mint leaves
> freshly ground black pepper

When you slice the cucumbers, leave the skin on half of them for color. Sprinkle with ¼ teaspoon salt and set aside in a colander for 20 minutes in a sink. This will allow excess water to drain from the cucumbers. After 20 minutes, press the liquid out of the cucumbers with a paper towel or a clean cloth. In a medium bowl, combine with the remaining ingredients and toss. Season with remaining salt and freshly ground pepper to taste.

Comforting Kale Salad

If desired, toss this salad with baked portabella mushrooms for a little extra oomph.

Combines with: Starch

Yield: 1–2 servings

> 1 bunch kale, stems and hard rims removed
> ½ teaspoon sea salt
> 1 to 2 tablespoons coconut aminos or freshly squeezed lemon juice
> ½ large avocado, halved
> ¼ cup chopped red onion
> ¼ cup nutritional yeast

In a large bowl, prepare the kale by tearing the leaves into smaller, bite-size pieces. Sprinkle with sea salt and toss. The sea salt will help the leaves absorb the flavor. Add the coconut aminos or lemon juice and avocado. Use your hands to massage the avocado oils into the leaves until all of the leaves are thoroughly coated and wilted. Add the remaining ingredients, toss, and serve.

Farmer's Bibb Salad

Combines with: Starch

Yield: 1–2 servings

> 2 heads Bibb lettuce, leaves separated and torn into pieces
> 1 (6-ounce) jar of hearts of palm, rinsed, drained, and cut into 1-inch rounds
> 1 avocado, halved and cubed
> ¼ cup diced shallots
> 1 tablespoon raw apple cider vinegar
> sea salt and freshly ground black pepper

Toss all the ingredients together, season to taste with salt and pepper, and serve.

Fennel Insalata

Combines with: Starch

Yield: 2 servings

  2 cups thinly shaved fennel bulb, cut on a mandoline
  ½ of a fresh squeezed lemon juice (about 1½ tablespoons)
  ⅛ teaspoon Himalayan sea salt
  2 garlic cloves, thinly shaved on a mandoline
  ¼ cup fresh parsley leaves
  ¼ cup fresh basil leaves
  ½ cup capers, rinsed
  1 avocado, cubed (optional)
  4 to 6 ounces arugula (optional)
  freshly ground black pepper

Toss all the ingredients together, except the arugula, and season with black pepper to taste. Serve on a bed of arugula, if using.

Glow Detox Kale Salad

Combines with: Starch

Yield: 1–2 servings

  1 bunch kale, stems and hard rims removed
  1 teaspoon sea salt
  2 to 3 tablespoons freshly squeezed lemon juice
  ½ large avocado, halved
  ¼ cup fresh parsley, chopped
  ¼ cup chopped scallions
  2 small garlic cloves, shaved or minced (optional)
  freshly ground black pepper
  red chili pepper flakes (optional)

In a large bowl, prepare the kale by tearing the leaves into smaller, bite-size pieces. Sprinkle with sea salt and toss. The sea salt will help the leaves absorb the flavor of the other ingredients. Add lemon juice and avocado. Then use your hands to massage the avocado oils into the leaves until all of the leaves are thoroughly coated and wilted. Add the remaining ingredients, seasoning to taste with black pepper and red chili pepper flakes, if using. Toss and serve.

Mediterranean Salad with Roasted Beets

Combines with: Neutral foods, Animal protein

Yield: 4–8 servings

> 12 medium beets
> 2 cups artichoke hearts
> ½ yellow onion, halved and thinly sliced on a mandoline
> 1 fennel bulb, thinly sliced on a mandoline (about 1½ cups)
> 1 tablespoon raw apple cider vinegar
> 1 tablespoon fresh lemon juice
> ⅛ teaspoon Himalayan sea salt
> 12 ounces mixed baby greens
> ½ cup raw sheep's Manchego, thinly sliced
> freshly ground black pepper

Preheat the oven to 375°F. Rinse the beets and trim the "roots." Place all the beets on a cookie sheet lined with parchment paper. Bake for 45 to 60 minutes, until beets are hissing with steam. The beets should be firm but still easily stabbed with a fork. Allow to cool for several minutes, or carefully run under running water with tongs. The skin should easily peel off. Use your fingers or a knife to cut away the skin. Let cool in the fridge, and then quarter or dice.

Combine all the ingredients, except the beets, baby greens, and cheese, in a large bowl and toss. Plate on individual dishes or place on a serving platter. Display the beets around the greens (or the greens will turn red, unless using golden beets). Sprinkle with Manchego cheese.

Country Club Salad

Combines with: Neutral foods, Starch

Yield: 2 servings

> 2 heads romaine, finely chopped
> ¼ cup thinly sliced red onion
> ½ cup peeled and diced cucumber
> ½ cup diced tomato
> 2 tablespoons Honey Mustard Dressing (page 157)
> ½ large avocado, cut into chunks (optional as starch addition)

Toss all ingredients in a medium mixing bowl and serve.

Dressings

Herb Pesto Dressing

Combines with: Starch

Yield: 1½ cups

> 2 garlic cloves, coarsely chopped
> ¾ cup avocado
> ⅛ cup raw apple cider vinegar
> 1 tablespoon fresh lemon juice
> 1 tablespoon fresh lime juice
> 2 tablespoons chopped chives
> 2 tablespoons chopped fresh mint leaves
> ¼ teaspoon Celtic sea salt

Combine all the ingredients in a high-speed blender and blend until creamy. Serve as you like over greens, or use as a dip for carrots and other raw vegetables like celery and red bell peppers. Store in an airtight glass jar for up to 5 days in the refrigerator.

Dijon Vinaigrette

Combines with: Neutral foods

Yield: about 1 cup dressing

½ Spanish or yellow onion
¼ cup plus 2 tablespoons raw apple cider vinegar
¼ cup Dijon mustard
4 teaspoons celery salt
freshly ground black pepper

Grate the onion on a cheese grater and combine the pulp and accompanying juice in a high-speed blender with the remaining ingredients. Season to taste with freshly ground black pepper. Store in an airtight glass jar for up to 5 days in the refrigerator.

Honey Mustard Dressing

Combines with: Neutral foods

Yield ⅓ cup

¼ cup organic stone ground mustard (no salt added)
1 tablespoon cold pressed olive oil
2 to 4 tablespoons water (depending on your preference for thickness)
2 tablespoons raw honey (or use stevia to taste)

Blend all ingredients in a small blender until creamy, or whisk together all ingredients in a small bowl. Store in the fridge in a sealed container, or jar for up to 1 week.

Sides

Roasted Cauliflower Migas

Combines with: Neutral foods

Yield: 4–6 servings

  1 large or 2 small cauliflowers, cut into florets (about 2½ pounds)
  ½ teaspoon sea salt
  2 tablespoons vegetable broth, low sodium
  1 bunch scallions, all white and greens chopped and separated
  3 large poblano peppers, halved, seeded, and chopped
  ½ tablespoon onion powder
  ½ tablespoon garlic powder
  1 tablespoon ground cumin
  ½ teaspoon ground turmeric
  3 tablespoons Dijon mustard
  1 cup fresh cilantro leaves, chopped
  ¼ cup nutritional yeast (optional)
  freshly ground black pepper

Preheat the oven to 350°F. On a baking sheet lined with parchment paper, a non-stick pan liner, or aluminum foil, spread the cauliflower florets and sprinkle with sea salt. Bake for 25 minutes, or until the edges are browning. While the cauliflower is baking, warm a skillet over medium-high heat and add a thin layer of broth. "Dry" sauté the white bulbs of the scallions with the peppers until the liquid is absorbed. Turn off the heat. Remove the cauliflower from the oven and let cool for 2 minutes. Quickly take a thick spatula or a potato masher and break up the florets into chunky pieces, like scrambled eggs. Turn on the heat under the skillet and add 1 tablespoon of the broth to the skillet. Add the cauliflower pieces, spices, and mustard. Add splashes of broth as needed to prevent sticking. When the cauliflower mixture is warm, stir in the cilantro and nutritional yeast, if using. Garnish with the green parts of the scallion. Season to taste with salt and pepper.

Curried Sweet Potatoes

Cooled sweet potatoes make for a tasty addition to salads.

Combines with: Starch

Yield: 1–2 servings

> 1 large sweet potato, peeled and cubed (about 1 pound)
> ⅛ teaspoon sea salt
> ½ teaspoon curry powder

Preheat the oven to 375°F. Toss the sweet potato cubes in a small bowl with the salt and curry. Bake for 25 to 30 minutes, or until the potatoes are wrinkling and the edges are browning. Bake for longer if you desire a crisper texture. Serve warm or cool and store in an airtight container for up to 3 days in the refrigerator.

Seasoned Shiitake Mushrooms

These mushrooms will have great flavor and become chewy while they are baking, making for an excellent meat alternative for salads and a delicious side.

Combines with: Neutral foods

Yield: 2–4 servings

> ½ pound shiitake mushrooms
> 1 tablespoon ground cumin
> 1 tablespoon ground coriander
> dusting of cayenne pepper
> sprinkle of sea salt

Preheat the oven to 375°F and line a baking sheet with parchment paper. Spread the mushrooms on the baking sheet and season with the cumin, coriander, cayenne, and salt. Bake for 10 to 12 minutes, or until crispy.

Miso-Glazed Eggplant

For a candida-free diet, use stevia rather than honey in this recipe.

Combines with: Starch

Yield: 2–4 servings

EGGPLANT

1 pound eggplant, peeled and cubed, about 2 medium eggplants

½ teaspoon sea salt

2 tablespoons chopped chives

MISO GLAZE

¼ cup mellow white miso

2 tablespoons fresh lemon juice

4 tablespoons gluten-free tamari

2 tablespoons raw honey or 14 drops liquid stevia

2 garlic cloves, minced

1 teaspoon grated fresh gingerroot

Preheat the oven to 400°F. Spread the eggplant cubes on a baking sheet lined with parchment paper, a non-stick pan liner, or aluminum and sprinkle with sea salt. Bake for 12 minutes, or until the edges are browning. While the eggplant is cooking, combine all the miso marinade ingredients in a high-speed blender and blend until smooth. Carefully remove the eggplant from the oven and transfer the cubes to a medium bowl. Toss with the miso glaze and garnish with chives to serve.

Roasted Golden Beets and Fennel in a Honey-Mustard Glaze

For a candida-free diet, use stevia rather than honey in this recipe.

Combines with: Neutral foods

Yield: 2–4 servings

> 4 medium to large golden beets (or 2 golden beets and 2 Chioggia beets for color)
> 1 large or 2 small fennel bulbs, quartered
> dash of sea salt, plus more to taste
> 3 tablespoons unsweetened mustard, like Dijon or stone-ground
> 2 tablespoons raw honey or 14 drops liquid stevia
> 1 tablespoon chopped fresh rosemary
> ¼ cup chopped fresh parsley leaves
> 1 tablespoon fresh lemon juice
> freshly ground black pepper, to taste

Preheat the oven to 400°F. Wrap the beets individually in foil. Place on a baking sheet and bake for 30 minutes on a medium-top oven rack. Line a second baking sheet with aluminum foil or parchment paper and lay out fennel pieces as if you were baking cookies. Sprinkle with a dash of sea salt and place in the oven on a rack below the beets. Allow the beets and fennel to cook for another 10 to 15 minutes. When done, the beets should be tender and the fennel sizzling and browned at the edges. If the fennel is not browning, remove the finished beets and transfer the fennel to the top rack for a few minutes.

In a small bowl, whisk together the mustard, honey or stevia, rosemary, parsley, and lemon juice and set to the side.

Unwrap the beets and let cool for 20 minutes, or carefully rinse under cool water. The beet skins should easily peel off, but be careful—beets hold heat! Discard the skins and quarter the beets. Toss the beets, fennel, and marinade together and transfer to a serving dish. Sprinkle with sea salt and black pepper to taste.

Roasted Cauliflower

Combines with: Neutral foods

Yield: 4–6 servings

> 1 large cauliflower, cut into florets
> ¼ teaspoon Himalayan sea salt

Preheat the oven to 375°F. Spread the cauliflower florets on a baking sheet lined with a non-stick pan liner, aluminum foil, or parchment paper and sprinkle with sea salt. Bake for 20 minutes, or until edges are browning. Carefully remove from the oven and serve.

Savory Baked Sweet Potatoes

You can also make this recipe with a variety of winter squashes, depending on your budget.

Combines with: Starch

Yield: 4–6 servings

> 1½ pounds sweet potatoes, peeled and cubed
> 1 cup red onion, thinly sliced
> 1 tablespoon ground cumin
> 1 tablespoon ground coriander
> ½ teaspoon sea salt
> ¼ cup sliced scallions
> ½ cup coarsely chopped fresh cilantro leaves

Preheat the oven to 450°F and line two large baking sheets with foil. Spread the sweet potato cubes on both sheets and layer the onion slices on top. Sprinkle with the cumin, coriander, and sea salt. Cook for 25 to 30 minutes, until browning and tender. Remove from the oven and transfer to a serving dish. Top with scallions and cilantro to serve.

Mediterranean Tabbouleh

Combines with: Starches, Grains

Yield: 6–8 servings

1 cup quinoa

2 cups water or low-sodium vegetable broth

3 tablespoons fresh lemon juice

2 large avocados, cubed

2 garlic cloves, finely minced

1 bunch minced scallions, white and green parts

1 cup chopped fresh mint leaves (about 1 bunch)

½ cup chopped fresh flat-leaf parsley (about 1 bunch)

2 cups halved cherry tomatoes

1 teaspoon Himalayan sea salt, plus more

1 teaspoon freshly ground black pepper

Cook the quinoa according to the box instructions. Allow quinoa to cool and then toss all the ingredients (omit the avocado if you are not planning on enjoying right away) in a large bowl. Season with additional salt and pepper to taste. Serve immediately. Store, without avocado, in a sealed container and refrigerate overnight.

Marinated Artichoke and Asparagus

Combines with: Neutral foods

Yield: 4–6 servings

1 bunch thin asparagus, hard bottoms snapped off, chopped into 1-inch pieces

½ pint cherry tomatoes, halved

1 cup chopped artichoke hearts, packed in water (air-sealed packaging, jarred or frozen and thawed, preferably not canned)

1 tablespoon chopped fresh parsley leaves

1 tablespoon chopped fresh tarragon leaves

1½ tablespoons minced shallots

1 teaspoon grated lemon zest (from about 1 lemon)

2 tablespoons raw apple cider vinegar

Combine all the ingredients in a large bowl and toss. Transfer to a container with a lid and store overnight in the refrigerator.

Entrees

Herb Pesto Spaghetti

This recipe calls for one of my favorite kitchen gadgets, the spiralizer, which can be purchased from Amazon.com or Williams-Sonoma. If you don't have one, use a vegetable peeler to julienne vegetables into long matchstick pieces.

Combines with: Starch

Yield: 2–4 servings

> 4 large zucchini, spiralized
> 4 ounces mâche greens or baby field greens
> 1 cup microgreens
> 2 tablespoons diced red onion
> 1 cup Herb Pesto Dressing (page 156)
> sea salt and freshly ground black pepper
> fresh mint and chives, for garnish

Toss the zucchini, greens, and onion in a mixing bowl. Pour the pesto dressing over the vegetables. Toss and season with sea salt and freshly ground black pepper to taste. Garnish with mint and chives to serve.

Cinnamon Bun Oatmeal Loaf

Combines with: Starch (not perfectly combined)

Yield: 10–14 generous servings

> 2 cups or 1 (14-ounce) can coconut milk
> ½ cup plus 2 tablespoons raw coconut butter
> 2 teaspoons of vanilla extract or vanilla liquid stevia (I like NuNaturals brand)
> ½ cup grade B maple syrup
> 2 cups unsweetened applesauce
> 8 cups organic rolled oats
> 1 teaspoon salt
> 1 to 2 teaspoons ground cinnamon

Preheat the oven to 375°F and grease 5 (4 x 6-inch) loaf pans with coconut oil or spray with cooking spray. Heat the coconut milk and coconut butter in a medium pot over low heat for 10 minutes. When the coconut bits are melted, stir the vanilla, maple syrup, and applesauce. Stir to combine well and remove from the heat. In a large bowl, combine the oats, salt, and cinnamon. Pour in the liquid ingredients and stir well to combine. Divide the mixture among the prepared loaf pans. The batter will not rise, so don't worry about saving too much space on top. Bake for 12 to 15 minutes, until edges are browning and loaves appear firm. Let cool until you can safely pop out each loaf. Serve warm or at room temperature.

Simple Pasta Marinara (Oil-Free)

Combines with: Starch, Neutral foods

Yield: about 2 cups

> ¾ cup chopped red onion
> ½ red bell pepper, diced
> 2 garlic cloves, coarsely chopped
> ⅛ teaspoon sea salt, plus additional salt as needed
> ¾ cup diced heirloom tomato
> ¼ cup mashed ripe avocado (oil-free, starch option), or 1 tablespoon olive oil (contains oil, neutral option)

Heat a medium pot over medium-high heat and add the onions, bell pepper, garlic, and salt. Stir frequently to prevent sticking for 2 minutes. Reduce the heat to low and add tomatoes. Stir for another 2 minutes, and cover for 5 minutes. When mixture is steaming, uncover and carefully scoop the ingredients into a high-speed blender or food processor. Blend or process until well combined and chunky. Add the avocado or olive oil and pulse again until smooth. The blending process actually continues to heat the sauce. If not ready to serve, pour mixture back into your pot, cover, and leave on low heat until ready to use.

Spicy Puttanesca Sauce

Combines with: Neutral foods

Yield: 8–12 servings

> ½ cup low-sodium vegetable broth
> 1 cup diced white onion
> 4 cloves garlic, minced
> ½ teaspoon crushed red chili pepper
> 1 tablespoon no-salt-added tomato paste
> 2 (28-ounce) cans whole tomatoes, drained and chopped
> or 4 cups diced plum tomatoes
> ¼ cup pitted kalamata olives, chopped
> 2 tablespoons capers, rinsed and drained
> 3 tablespoons chopped fresh basil
> 3 tablespoons chopped fresh curly parsley
> 2 tablespoons minced fresh oregano
> 16 ounces gluten-free pasta of choice or 8 large zucchini,
> julienned or spiralized or lightly steamed vegetables

Heat the broth to a simmer in a large skillet over medium heat. Add the onion, garlic, and crushed red pepper and cook for 4 minutes, or until the onions are translucent and beginning to brown. Stir in the tomato paste and cook for 1 minute, stirring. Add the tomatoes, olives, and capers, and bring to a simmer. Reduce the heat to medium and cook for 20 minutes, stirring occasionally. Remove from the heat and stir in the basil, parsley, and oregano. Serve over cooked gluten-free pasta, zucchini noodles, or lightly steamed vegetables.

Sweet Potato Noodles

Combines with: Starch

Yield: 6–8 servings

> vegetable broth or water, as needed
> 3 medium sweet potatoes, julienned or made into noo-
> dles with the spiralizer

1 large zucchini, julienned or made into noodles with the spiralizer
3 to 4 cups Roasted Red Pepper Coconut Curry Sauce (page 177) or 2 cups Simple Pasta Marinara (page 165)
Optional add-ins:
baked eggplant cubes
baked mushrooms
roasted cauliflower
roasted red peppers
frozen peas, thawed

Add just enough vegetable broth or water to coat the bottom of a large skillet or pan. Heat the skillet over medium heat and add the sweet potato noodles, cover the pan, and cook for 2 minutes. Toss in the zucchini noodles, and pour in the Roasted Red Pepper Coconut Curry Sauce or Simple Pasta Marinara. Cover and cook for another 30 seconds and add any additional veggies. Serve warm.

Greek Medina Burger

Combines with: Starch

Yield: 1 serving

1 large portabella mushroom
¼ teaspoon ground cumin
¼ teaspoon ground coriander
gluten-free sprouted English muffin or burger bun, toasted (optional)
¼ large ripe avocado
slice of red onion
4 Cerignola olives, pitted and halved (large, mild green olives)
2 tablespoons Eggplant Caviar (page 178)
⅛ cup organic arugula leaves
4 sun-dried tomatoes, rehydrated in water for 8 minutes and coarsely chopped

Preheat the oven to 375°F. Place the portabella mushroom gill-side up on a baking sheet lined with a non-stick pan liner, aluminum foil, or parchment paper and sprinkle with the cumin and coriander. Bake for 10 minutes, or until the mushroom's juices are pooling on top. Bake for longer if you desire a chewier texture. Toast the English muffin or burger bun, if using. Using a fork, mash the avocado into both sides of the toast. Place the onion slice and olives on the top half of the toast and press down. In a small bowl, whisk together the Eggplant Caviar, arugula, and sun-dried tomatoes. Place the baked mushroom gill-side up on the bottom half of the toast and scoop Eggplant Caviar mixture into the cavity. Carefully place the two halves together and enjoy. The more beautifying option is to enjoy this burger without bread on a giant salad. Choose a salad that combines with a starch in the salad category of this book beginning on page 149.

Bunless Cheese "Burger"

Serve your "burger" with a side of sautéed green beans or wax beans with ketchup for dipping. Note that a candida-free diet should exclude added sugars and vinegars, which includes many store-bought condiments. If you're eating candida-free, be sure to limit the condiments on your burger.

Combines with: Animal protein

Yield: 1–2 servings

    2 large portabella mushrooms, stems removed
    2 teaspoons ground cumin, divided
    2 teaspoons ground coriander
    1 tablespoon coconut aminos, divided
    ½ cup shredded raw goat's or sheep's milk cheese, or goat's milk feta
    3 cups chopped romaine lettuce, divided
    1 to 2 slices of onion

Condiments of choice: organic ketchup, no-sugar-added mustard, unpasteurized kimchi

Preheat the oven to 375°F. Place the portabella mushrooms gill-side up on a baking sheet, lined with a non-stick pan liner, aluminum foil, or parchment paper and sprinkle with the cumin and coriander. Drizzle the coconut aminos onto each mushroom cap. Bake for 10 minutes, or until the mushrooms' juices are pooling on top. Bake for longer if you desire a chewier texture. Set the mushrooms onto a dish and sprinkle with the cheese. Place each mushroom on chopped romaine and top with onion slices and condiments, if desired, to give yourself the "burger" feel.

Pan-Seared Ahi Tuna Teriyaki

Combines with: Animal protein

Yield: 2 servings

½ tablespoon unsalted butter
1 bunch scallions, white and green parts chopped
1 inch peeled gingerroot, chopped
2 garlic cloves, minced
2 (4-ounce) ahi tuna steaks
¼ cup gluten-free tamari or raw coconut aminos
2 tablespoons grade B maple syrup

In a medium skillet, melt the butter over medium heat, using a spatula to coat the bottom of the pan evenly. Lightly sauté the scallions, ginger, and garlic for 2 minutes. Increase the heat to medium-high and add the tuna steaks. Sear each side for 2 minutes, or to the desired doneness, adding the tamari or coconut aminos and maple syrup before flipping. The inside of each steak should be pink. Serve immediately.

The Fresh Pick "Pasta" Salad

Combines with: Raw foods, Starch

Yield: 4–6 servings

2 large zucchini, spiralized or julienned

1 large yellow summer squash, spiralized or julienned

⅛ teaspoon sea salt, plus more

2 large carrots, peeled and julienned

1 cup cherry tomatoes, halved

1 cup fresh or frozen and thawed green peas

4 asparagus spears, thinly sliced with a vegetable peeler

2 large garlic cloves, thinly sliced or finely chopped

½ cup basil, loosely packed, torn into small pieces

¼ cup fresh flat-leaf parsley, chopped

juice of ½ lemon

1 tablespoon raw apple cider vinegar

1 avocado, halved and cut into chunks (optional)

freshly ground black pepper

Place the prepared zucchini and yellow squash in a large bowl lined with a paper towel to absorb excess water. Sprinkle with sea salt. In a separate mixing bowl, combine the carrots, tomatoes, peas, asparagus, garlic, and herbs, and toss with the lemon juice, apple cider vinegar, and avocado, if using. Dab the excess water from the "noodles," using a new paper towel or cloth if necessary, then toss all ingredients until well integrated. Season with salt and pepper to taste.

Portabella Mushroom Steaks

Combines with: Neutral foods

Yield: 2–4 servings

4 large portabella mushrooms, stems removed

4 teaspoons ground cumin, divided

4 teaspoons ground coriander, divided

1 teaspoon smoked paprika, divided

sea salt

1 cup Roasted Garlic Chimichurri Sauce (page 179)

Preheat the oven to 375°F. Place the portabella mushrooms gill-side up on a baking sheet lined with a non-stick pan liner, aluminum foil, or parchment paper and sprinkle each with the cumin, coriander, and paprika. Each mushroom should receive a generous pinch. Bake for 10 minutes, or until the mushrooms' juices are pooling on top. Bake for longer if you desire a chewier texture. Remove from the oven and drizzle each mushroom with ¼ cup of Roasted Garlic Chimichurri Sauce. Serve immediately, or keep in the oven on warm.

Baked Eggplant Rollatini with Roasted Red Pepper Filling

Combines with: Neutral foods

Yield: 6–12 servings

EGGPLANT

4 medium-large eggplants, tops and bottom removed, sliced vertically into ½-centimeter-wide slices
20 basil leaves, chiffonaded, for garnish
freshly ground black pepper

ROASTED RED PEPPER FILLING

2 large eggplants, sliced into medallions
2 medium red bell peppers
2 garlic cloves
1 tablespoon raw coconut aminos
2 tablespoons nutritional yeast (optional)
¼ teaspoon Himalayan sea salt
freshly ground black pepper

Preheat the oven to 375°F. Lay out the long eggplant pieces on a baking sheet lined with parchment paper. Do the same with the eggplant medallions and then the bell peppers on a separate sheet. Bake the eggplants for 25 minutes, until they brown at the edges and shrivel in the center. Bake the peppers for about 40 minutes, until browning.

Peel the skin from the peppers and discard. Combine all the filling ingredients and blend until smooth. Lay out the long eggplant slices on a cutting board. Using a spoon, scoop a generous spoonful of the roasted red pepper filling onto each eggplant slice and spread it out like you are buttering toast. Starting at the end closest to you, use your finger to roll up each slice away from you. Once rolled, place on a serving dish. Repeat with the remaining strips. Finish with a layer of basil chiffonade and freshly ground pepper to taste.

Creamy Quick Kelp Noodles

Kelp noodles are thin "noodles" made from a type of seaweed—kelp. Unlike most "noodles," these have a unique, almost "bouncy" texture. They are also very mild in flavor and can be a good alternative for someone looking to avoid gluten and grain products. Kelp noodles are also a good source of iodine. Kelp noodles can be found in specialty health food grocers like Whole Foods Market and also online.

Combines with: Starch

Yield: 2–4 servings

> 12 ounces kelp noodles
> juice of ½ lemon
> 1 ripe avocado
> 1 garlic clove, finely minced
> 2 tablespoons finely chopped fresh cilantro
> pinch of salt, plus more
> 3 cups baby arugula, baby kale, finely chopped curly kale, or mixed greens
> freshly ground black pepper

Soak the kelp noodles in warm water for about 10 minutes. Drain and transfer to a dry bowl. Pat the noodles dry if needed.

Toss the noodles in the lemon juice and allow to soak while preparing the remaining ingredients. Combine the avocado, garlic, cilantro, and salt in a small bowl and use a fork to mash the ingredients together. Toss the kelp noodles with the greens and the avocado mixture. Use your hands to "massage" the avocado oils into the noodles and greens. Season to taste with pepper and additional salt, as needed.

Marinated Coconut Sashimi

Combines with: Starch

Yield: 1 serving

> 1 cup young Thai coconut meat (about one coconut), cut into skinny strips if necessary
> ⅛ teaspoon peeled, finely minced gingerroot
> ½ teaspoon finely minced garlic
> ¼ cup raw coconut aminos

Carefully open the coconut. Pour out the water into a container or cup and scoop out the white meat into a small bowl.

Prepare the marinade by pouring all the ingredients into a bowl and whisking together. Marinate the coconut meat overnight, or for at least 4 hours, in a covered bowl, container, or zip-top bag before serving. If time is of the essence, use marinade as a dressing or dipping sauce for coconut meat. Enjoy this "sashimi" as is or as part of a sushi roll.

Grain-Free Vegan Sushi

Combines with: Neutral foods, Starch

Yield: 5–10 servings

> SUSHI WRAPPER
> about 5 collard green leaves
> 10 nori wraps (1 to 2 per person)

IDEAS FOR FILLERS

shredded carrot

shredded beet

shredded zucchini

shredded daikon

green onions/chives, finely sliced

sunflower sprouts

onion or other sprouts

peeled and sliced cucumbers

red onion, sliced

assorted mixed greens

cilantro leaves

avocado, thinly sliced

Marinated Coconut Sashimi (page 173)

Remove the hard spines from the collard greens, and trim with a sharp knife so that they are approximately half the size of a nori wrapper. (About 2 strips per collard leaf, depending on size). Lay down 1 nori sheet and layer with a piece of collard green on the side closest to you. This is meant to "line" the nori wrapper to prevent it from getting soggy from the fillers, so it is only necessary to be where the fillers are.

Prepare a small cup of water for you to wet your fingers.

For a basic roll, choose a leafy green filler, sprouts, onion, a shredded vegetable, and avocado. (Or whatever you like, making sure it is not too hard to roll up.) Thoughtfully stack your selection of fillers on top of one another in a narrow line over the collard green, staying about 1 inch away from the edge closest to you. Fold the nori wrapper over the fillers and tightly roll the sheet away from you.

Wet your clean fingers with water and just barely dampen the edge of the nori wrapper so that it sticks to itself. Repeat. Using a serrated knife, hold each "roll" and carefully slice into 4 to 6 bite-size pieces.

Greek Omelet

For best digestion, serve this omelet over raw mixed greens with lightly steamed low-starch vegetables, like broccoli.

Combines with: Animal protein

Yield: 1 serving

> organic butter or cooking spray
> ¼ cup diced red or yellow onion
> ¼ cup diced fresh tomatoes
> 1 large handful organic spinach
> 2 tablespoons diced green olives (optional)
> 3 organic, free-range eggs
> 1 teaspoon salt-free Italian seasoning blend
> goat feta or sheep Manchego, to garnish

Heat a medium ceramic or nonstick skillet over medium-high heat and coat the pan with butter or cooking spray, if needed. Add the onion and tomatoes and quickly sauté until the onions are translucent, about 2 minutes. Add the spinach and olives, if using, and sauté for 1 minute. In a small bowl, beat the eggs with the seasoning blend and pour over the vegetables. Increase the heat to high and scramble the eggs until cooked through, or treat as an omelet, and flip when the eggs touching the edges of the pan have cooked. Garnish with a light sprinkle of cheese. Serve over a bed of mixed greens and a side of steamed low-starch vegetables.

Almond-Crusted Eggplant

Combines with: Nuts, seeds, and dried fruits

Yield: 4–6 servings

> 1 cup almond flour
> 1 teaspoon garlic powder
> 1 teaspoon paprika
> ¼ teaspoon sea salt
> 1 teaspoon freshly ground black pepper

1 cup almond milk, freshly made or store-bought

2 large eggplants, sliced into medallions

Simple Pasta Marinara Sauce (page 165), to serve
(optional)

Preheat oven to 375°F and line 2 baking sheets with a non-stick pan liner, aluminum foil, or parchment paper. In a bowl, mix the almond flour, garlic powder, paprika, salt, and pepper. Pour the almond milk into a shallow bowl. Dip one eggplant medallion into the almond milk, then into the almond flour mixture, and then lay it on the prepared cookie sheet. Repeat with the remaining eggplant medallions. Bake for 30 minutes, turning after about 15 minutes, until coating is golden brown and dry. Top with marinara sauce, if using, and serve hot.

Simple Nori Burrito

Combines with: Raw foods, Starch

Yield: 1 serving, or 2 wraps

1 collard green leaf

2 nori wraps

½ avocado, divided

½ cup chopped cilantro leaves

¼ teaspoon garlic powder, divided

⅛ teaspoon sea salt

freshly ground black pepper

Remove the hard spine from the collard green with a sharp knife and cut in half, trimming so the pieces are approximately half the size of a nori wrap. Lay down 1 nori sheet and layer with a collard green piece on the side closest to you. This is meant to "line" the nori to prevent it from getting soggy from the fillers, so it is only necessary to be where the fillers are.

Prepare a small cup of water for you to wet your fingers.

Gently mash the avocado onto the collard, in a horizontal line. Follow it with cilantro and spices, leaving about a 1-inch border from, the edge closest to you. Fold the nori wrap over the fillers and roll the sheet tightly away from you. Wet your clean fingers with water and just barely dampen the edge of the nori wrapper so that it sticks to itself. Repeat with the second nori wrap. Using a serrated knife, hold each "roll" and carefully slice into 4 to 6 bite-size pieces.

Dips and Sauces

Low-Fat Chunky Guacamole

Combines with: Starch

Yield: 5–8 generous servings

>   5 large ripe avocados, cubed
>   1 cup peeled, finely diced cucumber (about ½ large cucumber)
>   ¼ cup diced yellow onion
>   1 tablespoon coarsely chopped fresh cilantro
>   ¼ cup diced tomatoes or halved cherry tomatoes
>   1 jalapeño, seeded and finely chopped
>   2 garlic cloves, minced
>   1 tablespoon fresh lemon juice, or more
>   1 tablespoon fresh lime juice, or more
>   salt and freshly ground pepper

Scoop the avocado into a bowl and add the cucumber, onion, cilantro, tomatoes, jalapeño, and garlic. Use your hands or a spatula to toss and mix the ingredients until well combined. Add the lemon and lime juice, toss, and season with salt and pepper to taste.

Roasted Red Pepper Coconut Curry Sauce

For the coconut milk, I recommend using the meat of 1 young Thai coconut blended with pure water. The blending ratio is 1 cup of coconut meat to 1 cup of water. If you do not have access to a young Thai coconut, you can use 1 cup of canned coconut milk. Note that if you double this recipe, it can be stored in the fridge for up to 3 days and served as a vegetable dip.

Combines with: Starch

Yield: about 5 cups

> 1 to 4 tablespoons vegetable broth, for stir-frying
> 1 medium sweet potato, peeled and diced, about ½ a pound
> 2 large red bell peppers, diced
> 1 medium yellow onion, diced
> ½ teaspoon sea salt
>
> 1 cup unsweetened coconut milk
> 1½ teaspoons curry powder
> 1 tablespoon raw coconut aminos

Heat a skillet over high heat and add just enough vegetable broth to coat the bottom of the pan. Add the sweet potatoes, and cover the pan, allowing to steam for 1 minute. Remove the lid and add the peppers, onion, and sea salt. Cook, stirring, until the onion is translucent and the peppers are sweating, 4 to 6 minutes, adding broth as needed to prevent sticking. Transfer all the ingredients to a high-speed blender and add coconut milk, curry powder, and coconut aminos. Blend until smooth and serve over noodles and veggies.

Eggplant Caviar

Use this dip as a bean-free substitute for hummus or as a condiment on sandwiches and in salads.

Combines with: Neutral foods

Yield: 5 generous servings

> 30 roasted garlic cloves, coarsely chopped (about 2 bulbs)
> 2 (1-pound) globe eggplants, peeled and cubed
> 1 teaspoon finely grated lemon zest

1 to 2 tablespoons fresh lemon juice

1 tablespoon finely chopped fresh flat-leaf parsley

Preheat the oven to 375°F. Slice off the top of the garlic so that the tips of the cloves are exposed. Place on a baking sheet and bake for 45 minutes to 1 hour. The garlic should be browned on top and easily squeezed from their skins.

While the garlic is baking, lay out the eggplant on a baking sheet lined with a non-stick pan liner, aluminum foil, or parchment paper and bake for 18 to 20 minutes, until browned. Transfer the eggplant to a medium mixing bowl. Add the garlic and use a fork to roughly "puree" or mash. Add in the remaining ingredients and serve.

Roasted Garlic Chimichurri Sauce

Combines with: Starch, Neutral foods (without avocado)

Yield: about 1½ cups

about 15 large cloves or 2 to 3 small garlic heads (about ½ cup roasted and mashed)

½ cup avocado, mashed (or use ¼ cup olive oil as an alternative to avocado)

¼ cup fresh lemon juice

1 tablespoon raw apple cider vinegar

1 cup chopped fresh flat-leaf parsley

1 cup chopped fresh cilantro

¼ teaspoon dried oregano

1 tablespoon fresh thyme leaves

Preheat the oven to 375°F. Slice off the top of the garlic so that the tips of the cloves are exposed. Place on a baking sheet and bake for 45 minutes to 1 hour. The garlic should be browned on top and easily squeezed from their skins.

While the garlic is roasting, combine all the sauce ingredients in a high-speed blender and pulse. Carefully squeeze the roasted garlic into the mixture and blend until smooth. This sauce can be made in advance and stored in the refrigerator overnight.

Roasted Red Pepper Dipping Sauce

Combines with: Neutral foods

Yield: about 1 cup

   2 large red bell peppers
   ½ large yellow onion, sliced
   2 tablespoons raw coconut aminos or gluten-free tamari
   1 teaspoon garlic powder
   1 teaspoon wasabi powder (optional)

To roast the peppers, preheat the oven to 375°F and place the bell peppers on a baking sheet lined with a non-stick pan liner, aluminum foil, or parchment paper. Bake for 40 minutes, or until the peppers are wrinkling and browned on the top. While the peppers are baking, spread the onion slices on a second lined baking sheet and bake for 15 to 20 minutes, until the onions are sweating and browning at the edges. Remove the peppers and onions at their appropriate times and allow to cool down. Carefully peel the skin from the red peppers and place into a high-speed blender with the onions and remaining ingredients. Pulse until smooth and serve as a dipping sauce or salad dressing.

Entertaining

Tea Party "Crackers" and "Cheese"

Combines with: Nuts

Yield: 16 generous servings

   "CREAM CHEESE"
   1 cup macadamia nuts, soaked for 4 hours and drained
   1 cup cashews, soaked for 4 hours and drained
   2 garlic cloves
   1 cup fresh parsley
   2 tablespoons gluten-free tamari
   1½ tablespoons freshly squeezed lemon juice
   ¼ to ¾ cup water

"CRACKERS"

10 medium radishes, sliced thinly into medallions on a mandoline

¼ cup finely chopped chives

¼ teaspoon Celtic sea salt

Blend all of the cream cheese ingredients in a high-speed blender until smooth. Start with just ¼ cup water, only adding more if needed to help facilitate blending. Transfer the mixture into a sealable container and refrigerate for at least 2 hours. This is not a must but helps the "cheese" to solidify.

Spread each radish medallion with a teaspoon of "cream cheese" and lay flat on a serving platter. Sprinkle with chives and salt.

Barbecue Sauce

Combines with: Nuts, seeds, and dried fruit

Yield: 2 cups

1 cup sun-dried tomatoes, soaked in water for 8 minutes

½ red bell pepper, chopped

3 tablespoons coconut aminos

2 tablespoons raw apple cider vinegar

1 teaspoon smoked paprika

2 teaspoons ground cumin

1½ teaspoons chipotle powder

1 teaspoon chopped fresh garlic

⅛ teaspoon cayenne pepper

½ cup pitted dates, soaked until soft (about 2 hours)

Drain the sun-dried tomatoes and reserve ¼ cup of the soaking liquid. Blend all the ingredients in a high-speed blender until smooth, adding the reserved soaking liquid as needed (this should not be necessary with a high-speed blender). Transfer to a jar with a lid, and seal for up to 7 days.

Chipotle Sauce Variation: Follow the directions for Barbecue Sauce, but omit the dates.

California Barbecue Mushroom Steaks

Combines with: Neutral foods, Nuts

Yield: 10–12 servings

> 3 pounds portabella mushrooms, stems removed, thickly sliced
> 4 fresh sage leaves, coarsely chopped
> 4 fresh or dried bay leaves
> 4 garlic cloves, coarsely chopped
> 1 tablespoon dried thyme
> 5 tablespoons raw coconut aminos or gluten-free tamari
> 1 large bell red pepper, diced
> 3 stalks celery, diced
> 1 to 2 cups Barbecue Sauce (page 181)

Preheat the oven to 375°F. Spread the mushroom slices in a large casserole dish. Whisk all the remaining ingredients in a medium bowl and pour over mushrooms. If you are using barbecue sauce, let marinate for 30 minutes. Bake for 20 to 25 minutes, or until the mushrooms are browning and juicy (marinated mushrooms can bake for 10 to 15 minutes longer). After the mushrooms are done, carefully remove them from the oven and serve with the sauce or juices poured over them. You may place the casserole dish back into the oven on warm before serving.

Creamy Pea Dip

Combines with: Starch

Yield: 4–6 servings

> 16 ounces organic frozen peas, thawed for 20 minutes
> ¾ cup ripe avocado
> 4 teaspoons fresh lime juice
> 2 teaspoons minced garlic
> ⅛ teaspoon Celtic sea salt
> 2 cups water

freshly ground black pepper, to taste

2 tablespoons finely chopped chives, for garnish

Combine all the ingredients, except the chives, in a high-speed blender and blend until smooth. Sprinkle with chives for garnish. Enjoy as a chilled soup, a dip for vegetables, or in place of hummus. Add more water for a thinner consistency.

Dessert

Chocolate Avocado Mousse

If you suspect you may have candida, omit the dates.

Combines with: Starch

Yield: 4–6 servings

> 4 large avocados, halved
> ½ cup raw cacao
> ½ cup pitted dates, soaked in water for 2 hours (optional)
> 1 to 2 teaspoons vanilla liquid stevia (I recommend Alcohol-Free Vanilla Stevia by NuNaturals)

Place the avocado into the bowl of a food processor and process until smooth. Add 1 to 2 tablespoons water if needed to facilitate blending. If using dates, drain the soaking water. Add the remaining ingredients to the food processor and process until well combined and smooth. Scoop into 4 to 6 small serving dishes and refrigerate until ready to serve.

Gingered Banana Soft-Serve

Combines with: Starch, Nuts, seeds, and dried fruit, Fruit

Yield: 1–2 servings

> 2 frozen bananas, thawed for 4 minutes
> ½-inch piece fresh ginger, peeled and minced
> ½ teaspoon cinnamon

Combine all the ingredients in a high-speed blender and blend until creamy. Serve immediately.

Hot Cacao (Hot Chocolate)

Combines with: Starch

Yield: 1 cup

>   1 cup hot water
>   2 teaspoons raw cacao
>   14 drops liquid stevia, or to taste
>   ¼ cup almond or coconut milk (optional)

Bring the water to a boil and pour into a mug with cacao. Stir in the stevia until all ingredients are well combined. Then top with milk of choice. Enjoy hot!

Wolverine Trail Mix

This trail mix is packed with raw protein and raw fat. It's good source of vitamins, minerals, free-radical fighting antioxidants, and carbohydrates.

Combines with: Nuts, seeds, and dried fruit

Yield: 2½ cups or 20 (1-ounce) servings

>   ½ cup raw sunflower seeds
>   ½ cup raw pumpkin seeds
>   ¼ cup wolfberries (goji berries)
>   3 tablespoons unsweetened coconut flakes
>   ¼ cup raw cacao nibs
>   2 teaspoons raw honey
>   ⅛ teaspoon sea salt

Combine all the dry ingredients in a medium bowl, or a container with a lid, and toss until mixed. Add the honey and sea salt, and toss again, or cover with lid and shake until well mixed. Have on hand to enjoy for those "in-a-pinch" moments.

CHAPTER 9

Skincare Regimen Recommendations

Beautiful skin starts on the inside and radiates outward. When we eat a highly alkaline, whole plant-focused diet, we strengthen the immune system and nourish the skin from the inside. But don't do all of that work to smother your body in products that harm your skin from the outside. Make sure you give your skin the same love—inside and out.

Much of the beauty industry and product hype is a result of misleading marketing and "high dollar" advertising and phrasing. Do any of these trendy phrases sound familiar?

- "Reverse Aging"
- "New Age-Defying Formula"
- "Breakthrough Treatment"

The resulting "laboratory treatments" and "natural" products confuse their audience into thinking that synthetic fillers are nothing to think twice about, when in fact they further irritate the skin or become allergens.

The skin will absorb upward of 70 percent of what you put on it into your bloodstream. Therefore, products used on the skin to clean, moisturize, and "beautify" can be just as dangerous to the skin as the foods we eat.

Be on the lookout for common additives like parabens, phthalates, sodium lauryl sulfates, petrolatum, mineral oil, artificial colors, and the like. Unfortunately, just as we cannot buy our way to superior health, there is no beauty in a bottle. Consult www.ewg.org to determine the level of toxicity of your makeup and facial products.

Caring For Your Skin

Typically you will want to wash your face with a gentle, pH-balanced cleanser.

Infrared saunas, steam rooms, massages, and facials can be wonderful ways to remove toxins from the body. Be cautious of where you receive these treatments, especially facials. As mentioned above, the skin absorbs much of what is placed on it into the bloodstream. Even more importantly, however, are the harsh chemicals and "burning" peels some spas use for dramatic results. Pores can benefit from opening and cleansing techniques performed by trained professionals, but these treatments can also result in increased sensitivity and even scarring. I love facials, but make sure you don't just find the best deal in town. Research the types of products they use and get a feel for the facility. For example, personally, I would never get a facial from a nail salon.

THE SUN

I love the sun. One of the best sources of vitamin D is from the sun's ultraviolet rays, hence why vitamin D is often referred to as the "sunshine" vitamin.

Vitamin D is thought to have both vitamin and hormonal properties. It plays a role in strengthening the immune system, our bones and teeth, our muscles, and promotes a healthy heart and thyroid. Vitamin D also aids in absorbing calcium, one of the most alkaline minerals in the body. When any of these systems are compromised, the whole body is compromised. This extra stress on our organs indirectly compromises our skin.

Sunscreen blocks the skin from the sun's UV rays, which then prevents our bodies from synthesizing vitamin D. I believe that we all could use at least 10 to 15 minutes of bare-skin exposure to sunshine, during the middle of the day, every day. The amount of time in the sun will vary depending on your skin's pigmentation. Lighter individuals need less exposure to the sun than someone of much darker skin.

Of course, it is not wise to bask in the sun without protection, but one must be wary of sunscreen. Most traditional sunscreens contain highly toxic ingredients such as benzophenone, disodium EDTA, padimate O, and oxybenzone. Ironically, these damaging chemicals can actually age the skin and weaken our system to disease.

If you are going to be out in the sun for longer than 10 minutes, always bring a wide-brimmed hat. The sun is strongest between 10 a.m. and 2 p.m. In some places close to the equator, the sun is still strong even two hours later. This means that if you plan to be outdoors, try to plan your activities before 10 am. and after 2 p.m.

Diet also plays a large role in your sensitivity to the sun and heat. A diet rich in leafy greens, fruits, and vegetables will not only decrease body temperature and help you tolerate hotter temperatures, but also help to reverse the sun's damage. These mineral-rich foods provide the body with a hefty source of antioxidants that works to neutralize free radicals. Damaging chemicals found in traditional sunscreens can have the opposite effect, causing free radical formation, which speeds the aging process.

I also believe that the sun is a great healer and source of energy. The more toxic a person is, the less they can tolerate the heat. The more toxic our diets become, the less tolerant newer generations are to sunlight and heat. If you find that you are intolerant of the heat, expect this to change as you change your lifestyle.

Tanning beds are not the same as sunshine. Tanning beds are synthetic forms of ultraviolet rays that enhance signs of aging. Frequent tanners will notice a decrease in their skin's elasticity, more wrinkles, and age spots. In addition, the penetration of these sunlamps actually damages your body's ability to create collagen. Without collagen, the body cannot repair itself.

Exercise for Beautiful Skin

Exercise should be a part of every healthy living plan, including one for radiant skin. Although generally considered a solution for weight loss, it actually accelerates the detoxification of the body. Fewer toxins leads to a more beautiful and glowing complexion.

Benefits of Exercise for Beautiful Skin

- Exercise increases blood and lymph circulation. Blood and lymphatic fluids distribute essential nutrients to your cells and rid the body of toxic wastes.
- Toxins are released through the skin's pores when you sweat. There is an increase of toxins released during increased activity.
- Deep breathing provides the body with more oxygen, essential to the body's optimal performance. Carbon dioxide is a byproduct of the various functions performed by the body. More carbon dioxide is released as you exhale rapidly during more strenuous forms of exercise.
- Exercise decreases cortisol levels (considered a "stress hormone") and increases "feel-good" endorphins, or chemicals, giving your mood a natural boost. Positive energy can

transform a dull complexion, where as stress accelerates aging and may contribute to acne and other skin issues.

- The body stores toxins in the fatty tissue. Regular exercise decreases fat, giving the body fewer places to hold waste.
- Thinner people with acid-forming diets could be at more risk for aged skin and acne, as the body will store less and potentially harm the cells that keep us looking youthful, or eliminate more toxins through the pores. While exercise is an excellent detoxifier, the body needs to receive the appropriate alkaline fuel to energize and refuel in order to prevent premature aging and skin issues.

Additional Exercise Tips

- All forms of exercise can be beneficial in appropriate amounts. This simply means that overexercise, or regularly pushing the body to a point of stress and exhaustion, does not produce a favorable outcome, but daily, moderate exercise can be mood- and life-enhancing. Strive to get at least 30 minutes of exercise a day. I personally like the elliptical machine, running, and at least two heart-pumping exercise classes, twice weekly.
- Does exercise make you feel incredible? Step it up a notch and get involved in a daily heart-pumping exercise class. Just do not go over that amount.
- When you sweat, you are releasing toxins from the body through your pores. Be sure you use a clean towel to wipe away sweat, and be sure to shower after you finish up. If you are touching publicly used equipment, wash your hands with a sanitizer or soap and water between workouts. This will help you avoid transferring germs to your body and face.

- If you plan to use a steam room after a sweat, rinse before going in.
- If you are one to shower at the gym, note what type of products they are using. To save money, some workout facilities will use low-quality products that can cause skin irritation. In doubt? Bring your own!
- Chlorine is one of the ten highest-volume chemicals made in the United States. It is commonly used to disinfect pools, hot tubs, and saunas, and it is used in most household cleaning products. Though we come in contact with chlorine far more than we think (potentially while showering and in drinking water), it becomes a particular issue for swimmers. As far as swimming pools and hot tubs go, chlorine can offset the skin's balance. Because the skin absorbs what is placed on it, regularly swimming or soaking in chlorinated bodies of water is not beauty-enhancing, as chlorine strips the body of its natural oils and can cause your skin to look dry and aged. In addition, as chlorine enters the body, it produces a corrosive acid that is damaging to the cells. Luckily, many gym facilities are moving towards salt-water pools, so if you are looking to join a gym, be sure to ask about their swimming facilities. If you find yourself without a choice, be sure to shower immediately after.

CHAPTER 10

Conclusion

Look in the mirror.

If you could turn back the clock and go back in time, what words of wisdom would you offer your newly educated self? What advice would you give before you had blemishes or wrinkles and before you started to notice the little things you wished you could will away with a cream, procedure, or pill?

It's not too late to experience your most beautiful skin now. While we cannot go back in time, we can most certainly begin to reverse the damage that we see in our reflection today.

When I was in the seventh grade, the worst—and looking back, the "best"—thing happened to me: a rosy blemish appeared on my chin. Adhering to the advice I was given, I diligently dabbed it with rubbing alcohol—the drying effect was supposed to eliminate all signs of its ugliness. Unfortunately, this did little to help the goal I was ultimately seeking: beautiful skin. In fact, it only aggravated the area, inflaming it so that it made my soft and youthful skin dry and red, in addition to being bumpy. Of course, no matter what defense I chose as my armor, none of them seemed to be the solution.

A decade later, I was still struggling through imperfections, misdirection, and misadvise. I now deem those little issues (which later turned into much *worse* inflammation, acne, wrinkles, uneven skin tone, and even scarring) blessings in disguise. My distress forced me to search beyond topical remedies, prescriptions, and procedures, and discover a solution that I could share with the world.

The good news is, as you reduce the clutter and baggage you have accumulated from within, and start to free up the energy otherwise diverted to internal stress, you can focus your new energy elsewhere and fully enjoy the blessing of your naturally radiant, youthful, and glowing complexion, which will far surpass the temporary relief you may receive from any other topical or invasive procedure.

Beautiful skin begins on the inside and radiates outward, which means this places the power in your own hands. What you put in (and on) your body—food, beverages, makeup, chemicals, lotions, medicine, perfume, thoughts (negative and positive)—and what you take out of your body are the solution to a radiant and clear complexion at any age.

I cannot wait to hear the success stories from all of you, as you discover your most beautiful complexion. Remember:

- Focus.
- Nourish your body.
- Hydrate your body with water from a good source.
- Alkalize the existing acidity and focus on alkalizing foods (greens, vegetables, etc.). The more water-containing fruits and vegetables you eat, the less water your body needs.
- Get exercise and ease stress.
- Eliminate, eliminate, eliminate. Let the waste go.

Appendix

Food Combining

Here is a break down of each food group as well as a quick reference chart.

Fresh Fruit: Should be limited to your morning meal, following a green juice or green smoothie. Bananas are exceptions to the rule and may be combined with nuts, seeds, dried fruit, and starches.

Vegetables: Enjoy with all categories of food for increased nutrients, fiber, and hydration. This column should be the focal point of your diet for beautiful, youthful, radiant skin. These groups are loosely listed in order of their alkalinity. Generally, the longer a food is heated, the less alkaline it becomes and the less nutrients and enzymes it will have to promote cell regeneration.

Starches: Every item listed under the starch category is designed to help paint a picture of what foods are considered starches, including examples of each. This category is best consumed with an abundance of low-starch vegetables.

Legumes: Legumes are a challenging food to digest regardless of how they are combined. Sprouted legumes are the easiest to digest. For the sake of combining, legumes should be eaten with an abundance of leafy greens and vegetables, but can be eaten with starches as well for flavor.

Nuts, Seeds, and Dried Fruits: Always look for raw or raw-sprouted nut and seed varieties. Steer clear of roasted, salted, and oiled varieties. This category, because already rich in fat and challenging to digest, should be eaten with leafy greens and raw vegetables and kept separate from meals.

Animal Proteins: Animal proteins should only be enjoyed with low-starch vegetables. It is best not to eat a variety of meats at once. For optimal digestion and beautiful skin, choose one animal protein and balance it out with an abundance of leafy greens and low-starch vegetables. If not choosing cheese as your "main" protein, a little raw goat or sheep cheese can be used to enhance a dish's flavor.

Food Combining

Green Juices and Smoothies *Enjoy alone on an empty stomach prior to eating*	· See pages 142–147 for recipe ideas		
Fresh Fruit *Enjoy alone on an empty stomach as a "breakfast" or morning meal*	· See page 87 for subcategories of fruit		
Starches *Enjoy with vegetable category*	· Avocados · Young coconut meat · Potatoes (all varieties) **High-Starch Veggies:** · Cooked corn · Peas · Cooked carrots	**Gluten-Free Grains:** · Amaranth · Buckwheat · Millet · Quinoa · Oats · Brown rice · Avocados · Young coconut meat	**Winter Squash:** · Spaghetti · Acorn, etc. **Grains (with gluten):** · Kamut, spelt, wheat, etc. · Bread **Legumes:** · Difficult to digest alone, best consumed with limited starches and an abundance of low-starch vegetables

Food Combining

Nuts, Seeds, and Dried Fruit *Best enjoyed with leafy greens*	· Raw nuts* (all varieties) · Raw seeds (all varieties) · Dried fruit (unsweetened)	· Mature coconut (shredded coconut) · Nut/seed butters* · Bananas (an exception to the rule)	*Peanuts are not nuts, but legumes. They are highly acid-forming so they are not included.
Vegetables (low-starch) *Also considered neutral, enjoy with any category*	**Leafy Greens:** · Arugula · Baby kale · Baby romaine · Bok choy · Collards · Kale · Mâche · Mixed baby greens · Romaine · Spinach · Fresh herbs (cilantro, parsley, basil), etc. **Raw Veggies:** · Bell peppers (except green)	· Cherry tomatoes · Tomatoes · Julienned or shredded veggies · Raw corn · Hot peppers · Sun-dried tomatoes · Sprouts (all varieties) · Raw garlic **Lightly Steamed:** · Broccoli · Cauliflower · Zucchini · Summer squash	**Cooked:** · Artichokes · Roasted cauliflower · Roasted beets **Roasted or Baked:** · Zucchini · Eggplant · Mushrooms (excluding white button) · Garlic
Animal Protein *Enjoy with "Vegetables (low-starch)"*	· Eggs · Cheese (goat or sheep)	· Fish · Milk · Cream	· Yogurt · Meat
Neutral *Combines with ANY category*	· Vegetables (low-starch) · Lemons and limes · Coconut water · Dark chocolate	· Nut milks (almond, coconut, etc.) · Organic butter · Oils (excluding refined oils, soy, and canola)	**Olives:** · Castelvetrano olives · Cerignola olives

The pH of Common Foods

Very Alkaline	Moderately Alkaline	Low Alkaline	Very Low Alkaline
· Artichoke · Avocado · Asparagus · Broccoli · Cabbage · Carrots · Cauliflower · Celery · Chard · Cilantro · Collards · Eggplant · Endive · Fennel · Garlic · Ginger · Wheat grass · Leafy greens · Green beans · Jicama · Lemon · Onion · Radish · Sea vegetables · Seaweed · Squash · Sweet potato · Tomato · Zucchini · Lemon water · Herbal tea	· Almonds (raw, organic) · Buckwheat · Grouts · Burdock · Chia seeds · Cumin seeds · Flax seeds (raw) · Flax oil · Herbs (fresh) · Stevia · Sesame seeds (raw) · Sunflower seeds (raw, organic)	· Apples · Apricots · Bananas (ripe) · Blueberries · Cantaloupe · Cherries · Cold-pressed oils · Currants · Dates · Grapes · Kiwi · Mangos · Olive oil (expeller-pressed) · Oranges · Papayas · Pears · Pineapples · Plums · Pomegranates · Raspberries · Strawberries (organic) · Watermelon	· Carob · Herbs (dried) · Millet · Miso (organic) · Mushrooms · Pecans · Quinoa (organic) · Brown rice · Spelt · Vegetable broth · Walnuts · Wax beans · Vegetables, cooked · Wild rice

Neutral/ Near Neutral	Very Low Acid	Low Acid	Moderately Acid	Very Acid
· Butter (organic) · Coconut meat (young) · Coconut water · Water (source is important)	· Amaranth · Fish (wild, sustainable) · Dried fruit · Cooked fruit · Date sugar · Honey (raw) · Goat or sheep cheese (raw) · Lentils · Olives · Sprouted grains	· Barley · Rye · Cashews · Aged cheese · Corn oil · Cranberries · Granola · Legumes · Peanuts · Soybeans (processed, gmo) · Whole grains	· Bran · Bread · White flour · Chicken · Flour · Eggs · Cake · Corn meal · Crab · Lobster · Pasta · Pastries · Pork · White rice · Sausage · Shrimp · Turkey · Veal · Caffeinated teas (including green)	· Alcohol · Artificial sweetener · Candy · Cereal · Processed cheese · Cocoa · Coffee · Cottonseed oil · Milk (unless local) · Hydrogenated oil · Fried food · Ice cream · Jelly · Hops · Malt · Margarine · Msg · Processed foods · Pudding · Soda · Sugar · Table salt · Vegetable oil · Vinegar · Yeast

Be Social: Best Options When Dining Out

Being on the Clear Skin Detox Diet doesn't mean you can't be social. Here are some tips for dining at restaurants.

BEST SOCIAL BEVERAGES

- Herbal tea with stevia
- hot water with fresh lemon wedges
- red or white wine (sparkling wine not recommended)

DESSERTS

Desserts can be tempting so I suggest that you carry dark chocolate in your personal items. Or look for chocolates with at least 70% cacao content and no dairy on the menu.

Best Options When Dining Out

	Italian	Japanese/Asian	Mexican	Greek/ Mediterranean
Always to Start	Green salad with lemon, olive oil on the side, and freshly grated Parmesan cheese (optional). You can also just ask for a side of tomatoes!	Green salad with dressing on the side; if possible just ask for plain sesame oil on the side	Green salad with pico de gallo	Green salad with tomatoes, cucumbers, and olives
App A	Shrimp cocktail or mussels	Miso soup and sashimi with no rice	Guacamole with vegetable crudité; if steering clear of avocado, ask for salsa instead or skip to the entrée	Tomato and feta salad

Best Options When Dining Out

	Italian	Japanese/Asian	Mexican	Greek/Mediterranean
Entrée A	Baked fish with a side of steamed or lightly sautéed vegetables, plus a side of marinara sauce topped with Parmesan cheese	Baked with a side of steamed or lightly sautéed vegetables flavored with soy sauce OR a giant sashimi platter (no rice) with daikon noodles and steamed veggies	Giant salad in a corn tostada topped with pico de gallo and a side of steamed vegetables; add guacamole if eating avocado	Baked fish or chicken with a side of steamed or lightly sautéed vegetables; flavor with minimal butter
App B	Minestrone or other tomato-based soup	Miso soup and edamame	Make your own dish: order a side salad with fajita veggies; don't be afraid to bring along your own raw goat's/sheep's cheese	Hummus and vegetable crudités with olives, baba ghanoush, and olive spread
Entrée B	Whole wheat pasta tossed in butter or marinara sauce with a large side of steamed vegetables (no meat, fish, or cream)	Steamed vegetable platter with sautéed mushrooms; toss with soy sauce and order more edamame	Fish tacos without the tortilla or toppings: baked or broiled fish with a large side of vegetables or steamed broccoli	Vegetable dish with quinoa or potato dish (gluten-free), tabbouleh, couscous, or whole-wheat pasta (all contain gluten) Avoid meat and animal products
Other Notes	App B works well with both entrée options; the BEST entrée is always a big dish of steamed veggies with marinara sauce and Parmesan cheese (optional)		Most restaurants have a vegetable fajita option; you can easily order the veggies without the tortillas and toppings	

General Grocery Shopping List

Alternatives to Dairy and Soy Milk
- ☐ Almond milk
- ☐ Coconut milk
- ☐ Cashew milk
- ☐ Sunflower seed milk
- ☐ Hazelnut milk

Avoid: oat, rice, soy, and animal milks (cow, sheep, goat)

Cheese Alternatives
- ☐ Raw sheep's milk cheese, preferably unpasteurized
- ☐ Raw goat's milk cheese, preferably unpasteurized
- ☐ Pasteurized goat's milk or sheep's milk cheese .

Avoid: cow milk (both pasteurized and raw)

Alternatives to Peanut Butter
- ☐ Raw tahini
- ☐ Raw almond butter
- ☐ Sunbutter (sunflower seed butter)
- ☐ Alternative nut and seed butters, preferably raw

Bread, Tortillas, Bagels, and English Muffins
- ☐ Whole grain sprouted breads (freezer section)
- ☐ Ezekiel breads by Food For Life
- ☐ Breads from Alvarado Street Bakery
- ☐ Gluten-free sprouted bread

Pasta
- ☐ Organic corn and quinoa-based
- ☐ Gluten-free organic brown rice pasta
- ☐ Zucchini, julienned (preferable)

Alternative Sweeteners

- ❐ Liquid stevia without vegetable glycerin
- ❐ Raw honey, not pasteurized

Snacks

- ❐ Dehydrated fruit or veggies
- ❐ Dried fruit, unsulphured (raisins, mango)
- ❐ Raw nuts (not roasted, salted, or with added oil)
- ❐ Organic corn chips
- ❐ Organic popped chips
- ❐ Corn and pea-based chips (organic is ideal)
- ❐ Seaweed snacks
- ❐ Rice cakes
- ❐ Kamut cakes
- ❐ Spelt puffed cakes

Tip: look for baked chips

Cereal

- ❐ Gluten-free rice cereal
- ❐ Corn flakes
- ❐ Raw granola
- ❐ Cream of buckwheat
- ❐ Steel cut oats

Rice and Rice Alternatives

- ❐ Quinoa, all varieties
- ❐ Brown rice

Condiments and Sauces

- ❐ Raw salsa
- ❐ Salsa, without added vinegar
- ❐ Raw kimchi
- ❐ Fresh-made guacamole

- ☐ Organic ketchup
- ☐ Organic marinara sauce without soybean, canola oil, or added sugars
- ☐ Salt-free stone-ground mustard
- ☐ Raw coconut aminos
- ☐ Gluten-free tamari

Salt

- ☐ Pink Himalayan salt
- ☐ Celtic salt

Avoid: iodized salt

Olives

- ☐ Castelvetrano
- ☐ Cerignola
- ☐ Capers

Oils

- ☐ Olive oil, unfiltered, unrefined
- ☐ Raw coconut oil
- ☐ Raw coconut butter
- ☐ Organic butter, unsalted (OK to use for flavor and sautéing)

Avoid: canola, soy, and refined oils

Chocolate

- ☐ At least 70% and above, dairy-free, organic dark chocolate

Ice Cream Alternatives

- ☐ Coconut-based
- ☐ Goat-milk based

Avoid: cow, soy, and rice-based ice creams

Testimonies for Clear Skin Detox

Since embarking upon my journey to naturally clear skin, I have noticed few things that have made such an improvement as food combining, green juices, and cutting down on sugar. Food combining reduced about 90 percent of my breakouts and whiteheads, green juicing gave my skin a glow I've never experienced, and cutting down on sugar keeps my skin vibrant and keeps pimples from popping up. These three habits integrated as a part of my daily lifestyle have not only helped me achieve a beautiful complexion, but have also helped me feel comfortable and happy with what I see in the mirror.

—Jamie Leedom

I had severe eczema before beginning a detox lifestyle. I had open wounds all over my arms, coupled with large inflamed welts on my legs, back, torso, and even my face! My old doctor put me on some sort of "anti-fungal" drug that didn't help at all. I remember her disclaimer that she would only give me a two-week prescription because she didn't want to damage my liver...yikes!

I was extremely frustrated with the lack of real care I received. Aside from the scary prescription drug, her only advice was that I switch to a new brand of lotion. Neither helped much.

After the first few months of food combining, incorporating more raw foods, and colon cleansing, my skin cleared drastically. It was about a year into it that my skin had completely transformed from a nightmare to a dream! I have beautiful skin these days, and all I use on it is natural soap and coconut oil.

—Audrey Benevedes

I have seen a big difference in the clarity of my skin. My face and chest have really cleared up! I feel so thankful to have met Lauren and I am so encouraged by her wealth of knowledge!

—Maddie S.

I have lost 22 pounds and I feel better than ever. My skin has cleared up and my mood has been better ever since. It is way different from mainstream dieting because it is something I think I will stick with for the rest of my life.

—Alexa L.

I am so grateful to have found you and your program. This year I will turn 45 and I finally feel that I know how to take care of body in the best way possible. I feel younger, lighter, and energized. It's the perfect complement to my yoga practice and has taken it to new heights of awareness. My students keep asking me what I'm doing to keep my body trim and slim and my skin youthful and glowing. Thank you!

—Karen Buckner, Owner of Bikram Yoga Dallas

Since I began starting my day with green juice, and got rid of processed foods and most coffee, everyone I know either asks me if I've lost weight or if I've had work done. I can't remember having this much energy at any age.

—Bonnie Hearn Hill, author of *Killer Body*

Index

Acknowledgments

I would like to acknowledge the influential people in my life, without whom I would have chosen a more traditional path.

Cliché as it may be, my mother has always been my best friend. Whether it was a broken heart, a zit, a hard day, or just wanting to share the most ridiculous and comical story of the moment, my mother has always made me a priority in her life. I do not think I can ever thank her enough for devoting her time and love to me, nor can I fully express my appreciation for her genuine belief that I should reach for the stars.

Despite our differing opinions in the health and wellness fields, I have always been my father's daughter. Our differences have challenged me to seek greatness in my abilities and myself. Because of my dad's own hard work and dedication to provide for his family, I was able to receive an excellent college education. Most of all, my dad also inspired me to create and dream. From the stories he told me at bedtime, to the goals he painstakingly had me write down and visualize for myself, I am eternally grateful.

My little sister is one of the most amazing people I know. Her glowing personality and ability to make light of any situation makes life a joy. Thank you for always being proud of me and encouraging me in this work. I could not be more proud of you, and now I am so excited that you will be pursuing a degree in nutrition.

My little brother, Lee, is one of the hardest workers I know. His encouragement has kept me reaching for those stars, regardless of adversity. Lee, I appreciate you asking those "hard questions" to keep me focused and for being a listening ear for those moments of uncertainty.

Kristen—my best friend in the entire world. It goes without saying that life would be terrible without you. Thank you for always understanding me, embracing my quirky sense of humor, and accepting me despite my ability to stray from traditional nutritional beliefs. I have been so blessed to have you in my life. Despite our time and distance apart, knowing that we have each other's back makes my world a brighter place.

Tracey—this book would be incomplete without acknowledging you and the entire Kurland family: Shelia, Stan, Ashley, and Lauren. One of the most generous and loving families I know, you are all exceptional role models in so many inspiring ways. Thank you for loving me and for helping me to realize that everyone deserves to be loved.

Mary Wood—thank you for daring me to jump. You were a welcome catalyst for change in my life. Thank you for all those moments of laughter. You are a wonderful friend.

Brian Sommer—my story began far before we met, and it continues with you. Thank you for loving me, especially despite the fact that your culinary training and my passion for plant-based eating, are quite dissimilar. This might be bad for your image but you make the most incredible plant-based cuisine and you motivate me to create incredible dishes and to be the very best. Also to Jack, Chase, and Alissa, who continually test my nutritional knowledge and force me out of my comfort zone in the kitchen and in life. Thank you for helping me to grow and adapt as a chef, nutritionist, and step-mother. Without you three, I would not have the real life experience I need to relate to my clients with children. Thank you for letting me into your lives.

My clients— you inspire me daily. Because of you all, I am a better person every day. You challenge me to be more creative, accepting, loving, open, and full of life and wonder. Thank you so much for giving me the opportunity to serve you on your path to health, happiness, and beauty. I learn from each of you. As a guide, my life has a greater meaning. You challenge me to continually grow.

Finally, I must acknowledge Natalia Rose and the Detox World team. I am so grateful for the divine way your work came to me and for the amazing community you have built.

About the Author

A certified clinical nutritionist, **Lauren Talbot** came to this work after spending ten frustrating years in and out of spas and dermatology offices seeking the solution for a beautiful, blemish-free complexion. Lauren attributed her bad luck to genetics, trying everything from topical treatments to prescription remedies. It was not until discovering and then studying with celebrity nutritionist, Natalia Rose, CN, that she realized and understood the connection between diet and skin.

Lauren now works internationally with high-profile health- and beauty-conscious clients looking to discover the secrets and solution to a youthful, glowing and clear complexion, and overall health and wellness. Find her online at www.diaryofanutritionist.com and www.theglowdetoxdiet.com.